SEXUAL
AWARENESS

**Also by Barry and Emily McCarthy
available from Carroll & Graf**

Couple Sexual Awareness
Male Sexual Awareness

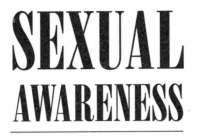

SEXUAL AWARENESS

UPDATED AND REVISED

COUPLE SEXUALITY
FOR THE
TWENTY-FIRST
CENTURY

ILLUSTRATED

BARRY AND EMILY McCARTHY

CARROLL & GRAF PUBLISHERS
NEW YORK

SEXUAL AWARENESS
COUPLE SEXUALITY FOR THE TWENTY-FIRST CENTURY

Carroll & Graf Publishers
An Imprint of Avalon Publishing Group Inc.
161 William Street, 16th Floor
New York, NY 10038

First Carroll & Graf trade paperback edition 1984
Second Carroll & Graf trade paperback edition 1993
Third Carroll & Graf trade paperback edition 2002

Library of Congress Cataloging-in-Publication Data is available.

ISBN: 0-7867-1015-2

Printed in the United States of America
Distributed by Publishers Group West

Contents

I

Introduction

1

Enhancing Sexual Awareness

There is a new sexual myth—almost all people are sexually knowledgeable and comfortable and sexual problems are rare. The scientific facts are that 50 percent of married couples and 65 percent of unmarried people report sexual dysfunction or dissatisfaction. Young couples have as many, if not more, sexual difficulties as older couples. The media is inundated with sexual material; people talk more openly and frequently about sex than ever before. Sexual experiences begin at a younger age. However, the sad fact is that sexual awareness, comfort, and satisfaction have *not* increased. The promises of the sexual revolution have not come true.

This book is designed to help people, especially couples, enhance sexual communication, feelings, and functioning. Our goal is to increase sexual awareness and comfort. We emphasize changing core sexual attitudes, behaviors, and feelings. We do not advocate esoteric procedures—you do not have to prove anything to yourself or to anyone else. The emphasis is on awareness, comfort, acceptance, and satisfaction rather than on performance or the necessity to prove you are sexually liberated.

Sexual intercourse is a core element of sexuality, but not the only, or even most important one. Sexuality is a positive, integral part of who you are as a person. Sexuality has not been appreciated as a healthy aspect of personality nor as an integral part of an intimate relationship. Sexuality is a source of excitement, jokes, and a symbol of adulthood, but it is also a source of conflict, guilt, and embarrassment about not being as sexually active and proficient as one's peers. Sexuality can and should enhance feelings about yourself and help you relate comfortably and intimately to another person.

Understanding and Accepting Sexuality

Healthy sexuality begins with understanding and accepting yourself, your body, and its sensual and sexual potential. In growing up there are two powerful negative teachings about sex. The first is that sex is basically bad (exciting, but bad) and becomes good only in the context of marriage. The second is that sex refers exclusively to intercourse. We believe that sex is a good thing in life and sexuality is an integral part of being a person. Sexuality is much more than intercourse. Sexuality includes everything from an affectionate glance to a gentle caress, from passionate intercourse to loving afterplay. The psychologically healthy question is how to express sexuality so that it enhances your self-esteem and increases satisfaction with your intimate relationship.

This is our fourth revision of *Sexual Awareness,* which was first published in 1975 and has sold over 500,000 books worldwide. There is a need for a book that addresses basic components of sexual awareness, comfort, and functioning. This book focuses on enhancing sexual attitudes, communication, and functioning, *but is not do-it-yourself sex therapy.* The exercises are meant to give the individual and couple an opportunity to learn healthy sexual scenarios and techniques. There is no requirement that all the exercises must be tried or that the reader must become proficient in a particular technique. Our hope is that the attitudes conveyed, the exercises described, and the feelings discussed will enhance acceptance, comfort, and sexual pleasure.

For individuals and couples experiencing a sexual dissatisfaction or dysfunction, this book is not a substitute for therapy. It is an aid in expanding sexual understanding and awareness. Marriage and sex therapists use these exercises as an adjunct in treatment. Section IV discusses the most common sexual problems. It will help you realize you are not alone in experiencing sexual difficulties and that these problems are resolvable. Appendix I presents guidelines for choosing an appropriate marital or sex therapist.

Another rationale for this book is to reach educational audiences, both college students and advanced students in the fields of psychology, medicine, marriage therapy, counseling, social work, health education, and the ministry. If students develop an awareness and comfort with sensuality and sexuality, their lives and the lives of clients with whom they work will be much improved. Education is the best means to prevent or remedy the harm that comes from sex myths, self-defeating attitudes, and negative experiences. This book is a step toward making sexuality a satisfying and positive part of life for the individual, couple, and culture.

Sources for Our View of Sexuality

The approach we utilize comes from two main sources: sex researchers (especially those engaged in social learning approaches) and sex therapists. Masters and Johnson were pioneers in the sex research and therapy fields. Their contributions have increased our knowledge of sexual behavior tremendously, both in the physiology of human sexual response and in treatment of sexual dysfunction. They dispelled myths which have caused damage to millions of men and women.

The social learning approach consists of strategies and techniques to help people learn new attitudes, skills, and emotional responses. Its premise is that the best way to learn or relearn healthy sexuality is through a gradual step-by-step method, assure one's comfort with the first experience before moving on to the next and through the utilization of supportive and constructive feedback to facilitate the learning process. The optimal condition for sexual awareness is commitment to an intimate relationship.

Who We Are

Emily and Barry McCarthy have spent over two years revising this manuscript. They have spent thirty-five years building a marital bond based on respect, trust, and intimacy and a vital sexual bond. In reviewing research, conducting marital and sex therapy, teaching human sexuality, conducting sexual enhancement workshops, and thinking about our marriage, our belief in the validity of these concepts has grown.

It is crucial to set aside couple time and value your relationship. Intimacy and non-demand pleasuring is the bedrock of sexual desire. The key to sexual arousal is erotic scenarios and techniques with one partner's arousal increasing and building on the other's. It is vital to reduce performance anxiety and replace unrealistic expectations with a pleasure-oriented, flexible, broad-based view of couple sexuality. This book offers strategies and techniques to help couples develop an intimate sexual relationship, which enhances satisfaction and stability.

This is the seventh book we have collaborated on. Barry is a practicing PhD clinical psychologist and a certified marital and sex therapist. Emily has a background in speech communication. We believe in these guidelines theoretically, clinically, and personally. We have found this book a pleasure to write and hope you find it worthwhile and valuable in enhancing your sexual awareness.

Comfort and Pleasure

We do not present specific exercises for sexual intercourse until chapter nine. Couples put too much emphasis on intercourse; this interferes with their full expression of sexuality. If a couple is comfortable with themselves and each other, feelings of sensuality, and their ability to give and receive pleasure-oriented touching, then intercourse and orgasm is a natural culmination of the sexual activity. Throughout the book there is consistent emphasis on *slow, gentle, tender, caring, rhythmic,* and *flowing* touching. These are essential ingredients for sexual satisfaction. When these are present during pleasuring/foreplay, in intercourse, and with afterplay, couples have increased satisfaction and enjoyment. An intimate relationship, non-demand pleasuring, and erotic stimulation are the core ingredients in sexual satisfaction, not esoteric techniques or acrobatic positions.

Couples Who Would Benefit from Marital or Sex Therapy

Couples experiencing severe conflict or communication difficulties, major individual psychological problems, or chronic sexual dysfunction will profit from seeking professional therapy rather than solely relying on these exercises. Couples who find marital or sex therapy effective are those in relationships in which one partner is enthusiastic and the other hesitant, in which both feel that having a professional third person would help the change process, or one in which both prefer to develop an individualized approach to their relationship and sexual problems. Maintaining motivation is one of the hardest elements in a self-help program. Being in therapy helps you deal with ambivalence, impasses, and disappointment. Guidelines for choosing a competent marital or sex therapist are presented in Appendix I.

Medical Factors in Assessment

When there is a question of physical or medical causes of sexual dysfunction, the ideal referral is to a physician with a sub-specialty in sexual medicine. Although the majority of sexual problems are not caused primarily by medical problems—exceptions being alcohol or drug abuse, uncontrolled diabetes, medication side effects, and chronic illness—it can be worthwhile to assess medical factors. Anything that impairs your general health can negatively impact sexuality. People typically begin with their internist or family practice physician, or the woman might consult a gynecologist and the man a urologist. Many physicians are not comfortable dealing with sexual issues, and try to quickly dispose of the problem by giving a prescription or making a joke. That is not what you want or need.

There is a growing trend to "medicalize" sexual problems. This was highlighted by the introduction of Viagra to treat erection problems in

1998. Our position is that Viagra, testosterone, estrogen replacements, and other medical interventions can be valuable resources in treating sexual dysfunction, but medical interventions alone are seldom the right answer for the complex psychological, relational, and sexual comfort and skill issues which are the core of couple sexuality. In the coming years there will be more pro-sexual medications, hormone treatments, creams, and patches which can be a valuable supplemental resource but must be integrated into the intimacy, pleasuring, and eroticism of the couple's sexual style.

HIV/AIDS and STDs

When we wrote the first edition of this book in 1975, the world had not heard of HIV/AIDS. How will this frightening reality (sex can cause death) affect sexual awareness?

Sexual comfort requires sexual health and safe sex. The safest sex involves couples who are intimate and committed, and who have tested negative for HIV and STDs (sexually transmitted diseases). This allows the full range of sexual experience and provides freedom from fear of contracting HIV or other STDs. Is that too idealistic? A new tradition among committed couples is to be tested for HIV and other STDs and to have an agreement of monogamy. The back-up is an agreement to inform the partner if one engages in any risky sexual activity with another person. If so, they will use a condom until they are retested. This involves trust in yourself and your partner, and is a solid base for comfortable, healthy sexuality.

When Barry first began teaching a college sexuality course in 1970, the main STDs were gonorrhea and syphilis. In the 1970s herpes (herpes simplex II) began to spread and became the most feared STD because it has no cure. Herpes was and is a serious STD that affects over forty million Americans. Now the most frequently contracted STDs are chlamydia and genital warts. However, all the STDs have been forgotten (which is not wise) with the furor over HIV/AIDS. This has dominated sexuality since the 1980s and will do so for the foreseeable future.

STDs and AIDS are not irrational fears. In their lifetime, approximately two out of five people will contract an STD. This needs to be dealt with as a health problem, not a moral judgement. The atmosphere of fear and stigma, viewing AIDS as God's revenge, and nature's way of halting sexuality, or as punishment for sexual excess, is counterproductive as well as untrue.

HIV (human immunodeficiency virus) is spread primarily through the mediums of blood, semen, and vaginal secretions. HIV is considerably easier to transmit sexually (as opposed to by blood or needles) by males (whether by heterosexual or homosexual contact), because semen is a more powerful medium for the virus than vaginal secretions. Vaginal and anal intercourse is more dangerous for the woman than the man. In other words, the transmission is most often from male to female or from male to male. Female to male transmission occurs, but is less likely. The exception is childbirth—females transmit HIV to their babies.

One of the scariest aspects of the epidemic is that the carriers of HIV are healthy people who have no symptoms and are usually unaware they are HIV positive. Once infected, the person stays infectious even though not ill. People with HIV eventually become ill with AIDS, but usually not for several years (the average is between eight and twelve).

So how can the person not in a monogamous relationship practice safe sex? The more aware, knowledgeable, and responsible you are about sexuality, the more you can protect your health against HIV/AIDS and other STDs. Unfortunately, like other STDs, HIV has a "sexist" bias. With gonorrhea, 90 percent of males are symptomatic, while only 25 percent of women are. The woman is therefore dependent on the man to be honest and to share the sensitive information that he is infected and she needs to be tested and treated. In the matter of HIV, the woman needs to be assertive in asking her partner whether he is "at risk" because of homosexual activity, IV drug use, or sex with prostitutes (the highest risk groups for HIV infection). However, be aware it is sexual behavior, not types of people, which spreads HIV. The best method is for both partners to be tested for HIV and other STDs and have an agreement to not be sexual with others—which means you have to trust that the partner will be honest if there is an incident. The second best preventative is to avoid activities involving exchange of semen and vaginal secretions. The highest risk activity is anal intercourse, followed by vaginal intercourse. Oral sex is less risky, especially if the male does not ejaculate into the woman's mouth. Some couples use condoms during fellatio or a dental dam during cunnilingus. The third preventative is to use condoms during intercourse—this is highly recommended for non-monogamous couples.

The most realistic criterion for judging sexual behavior is whether it is harmful to you or your relationship. This includes vulnerability to HIV, other STDs, unwanted pregnancy, physical pain, or psychological coercion. HIV/AIDS is a "sexist" disease; women are vulnerable to getting it from male partners. This is not to promote hysteria or paranoia, but to make both people aware that now more than ever it is crucial to establish respectful, trusting, and communicative relationships. Guidelines for healthy sexual behavior—to be aware, knowledgeable, caring, and responsible—will serve you well in dealing with STDs and HIV/AIDS.

The Concept of Exercises

These materials were originally developed in the context of sex therapy. In thirty years as a sex therapist, Barry has treated over two thousand couples. Barry sees couples for sex therapy sessions once a week. They have benefitted from structured exercises during the week to promote changing sexual attitudes, behavior, and feelings. We decided to utilize exercises independently of sex therapy when we realized many couples—particularly those who do not consider themselves candidates for sex therapy—could benefit from these exercises.

Couples can become comfortable communicating sexually by saying what feels good and what they want. Sexual dysfunction and dissatisfaction can be prevented by encouraging the couple to devote the time and psychological energy necessary to develop a couple's sexual style and to enhance their intimate relationship.

You are the best judge of whether our approach to enhancing sexual awareness and comfort will be helpful for you. If you decide marital or sex therapy would be more appropriate, we encourage you to seek professional therapy. You can use these exercises in conjunction with the therapist's suggestions. If undecided, you might read the chapter on non-genital touching and discuss it with your partner. We recommend you not to proceed with the exercises unless you and your partner have discussed expectations and agree to engage in the exercises in an involved, cooperative manner.

The Audience For This Book

People without regular partners are encouraged to read this book to increase their understanding and change their attitudes, but a good relationship is essential to benefit from the exercises themselves. It is better simply to read the material than attempt to use the exercises with someone with whom you are not comfortable, to whom you are not attracted, or whom you do not trust will be supportive of your sexual growth.

The exercises were written mainly (but not exclusively) with the married couple in mind—especially those husbands and wives who relate well but experience anxiety, inhibition, dissatisfaction, or dysfunction in their sexual relationship. These exercises have been used successfully by non-married couples who are committed to improving sexual communication and satisfaction. We have been particularly gratified to find the exercises used successfully by couples forty and older—they find these exercises help them reawaken and resensitize sensual and erotic feelings. Chapter 11 deals with sexual expression with aging (over sixty) and is particularly important because this is such a neglected area. People can function sexually into their sixties, seventies, and later. The idea that sex belongs to the young is one of the most cruel sex myths.

In addition, these exercises have been used by gay and lesbian couples. Although aimed toward heterosexual couples, these exercises are applicable to gays and lesbians with relatively few modifications. Of course, the exercises can be used by sexually well-functioning couples, since we can all benefit from enhancing sensual and sexual awareness.

In most chapters there is a case study. These are composite cases of clients Barry has seen in his practice, with names and details altered to protect confidentiality. The purpose of case studies is to make clear that "normal" people have sexual difficulties, to illustrate the variety of psychological, relational, and situational causes of sexual problems, and to offer reassurance that people can change and their sexual relationship can improve. The problems and solutions sound easy in a two-page summary, but, in fact, changing a couple's sexual pattern takes time and commitment, and is seldom a smooth, miraculous process.

Procedure for Exercises

We suggest the following procedure to facilitate using the exercises:

Begin by deciding what you want to learn about yourself and your partner.

Be aware that the best way to learn sexually is to understand your responses first, then give feedback and guide your partner. Among the best ways to give feedback are the following:

1. Be caring and constructive.
2. Give positive feedback before negative.
3. The best learning ratio is five positive to one negative.
4. Be specific, especially about requests for change.
5. When giving feedback, request the change you would like and avoid making negative comments about your partner as a person or lover.
6. Support your partner in making the changes you request.

Agree on how much time to spend on the exercises during the week; at least once a week is needed, twice a week would be better, and four times a week is ideal (seven times a week is overkill).

Exercises as Guidelines

The exercises should be regarded as guidelines rather than rigid, un-yielding rules. If you view the exercises as required homework or something you are forced to do, you will receive little enjoyment or benefit. Use exercises to help you explore, learn, accept, and increase comfort with sensual and sexual feelings. The exercises are meant to provide choices and alternatives so you can discover what you, indi-vidually and as part of a couple, find pleasurable and arousing. To en-hance sensual and sexual functioning, be spontaneous, try different techniques, share and communicate, and vary your approach. For in-stance, we emphasize the importance of slow, tender, gentle, rhythmic, flowing touching. However, if that is the only style of touching you use, it would become boring. At times, each partner would like rapid, in-tense, erotic touching. We suggest showering or bathing together, but you can also enjoy sex while being sweaty, as sensations can be en-hanced by natural body essences. Variety and experimentation are major ingredients in enhancing your sexual relationship.

How to Use These Exercises

Each chapter includes four sets of exercises. This fourfold division is intended to gradually increase comfort and skills. Feel free to move at your own pace; sensual and sexual feelings cannot be forced. Pushing too fast is a common problem. It is crucial that one partner not feel pressure to perform, so move at a comfortable pace.

The core of sexual awareness exercises consists of non-genital plea-suring (Chapter 3) and genital pleasuring (Chapter 4). Pleasuring enables you to increase awareness of sensual and sexual feelings, learn to be comfortable both giving and receiving pleasure, initiate and respond to sexual interactions, process feedback, and appreciate slow, gentle, tender, caring, rhythmic, flowing touching. Pleasure-oriented sexuality produces feelings of comfort, awareness, and intimacy, without which the exercises will lack value and can be counterproductive.

Avoiding Performance Orientation

We suggest you devote at least two weeks to the initial non-demand pleasuring exercises and, during that time, refrain from intercourse. So much sexual activity is goal-oriented and intercourse-oriented that sensual and sexual awareness is inhibited by the rush to intercourse and orgasm. Two weeks away from intercourse is well worth the effort to help you attain a solid sensual and sexual base. It is a worthwhile two-week investment in a sexual relationship that can be satisfying for years. In fact, we recommend that once a month or every other month, couples spend time in non-genital and genital pleasuring that does not culminate in intercourse. This reinforces awareness that not all touching is goal-directed. Intercourse is not the *only* means of sexual expression. Develop a variable, flexible, sensual and sexual repertoire and enjoy non–goal-oriented experiences.

During the weeks you are involved with non-genital and genital exercises, we suggest you engage in the self-exploration/masturbation exercises (Chapter 5) individually. Most men and women are neither as aware of nor as comfortable with their own body and sexual responses as they could be. Accepting your body's responsivity and orgasm triggers is the basis for sharing. Masturbation exercises can provide an orgasmic outlet during the period of non-demand exercises.

A good guideline for self-exploration exercises (and all other exercises) is to never do anything that causes you pain or is against your values. Do not proceed to the next step until you are comfortable with the preceding step. Remember, exercises are learning experiences.

Flexibility

Be as flexible as you wish in utilizing the exercises. We suggest you read through a chapter first by yourself. Then discuss it with your partner. Decide if and when you would like to proceed. Some couples go through each exercise step-by-step, while others combine two or more exercises or improvise as they go along. Decide what procedure is most comfortable for you.

We recommend you not do an exercise with the book open. This is not a cookbook. Sex requires two active, involved participants. For the exercises to be a positive learning and sharing experience, the most important ingredient is verbal and nonverbal feedback, because it is crucial to stay on the same intimate team and not get thrown off track by feelings of rejection, embarrassment, disappointment, or frustration. The exercises are flexible guidelines to enhance positive sexual attitudes, feelings, and functioning.

Communication

Communication is a key to sexual satisfaction. It is not easy to express one's feelings. After the first romantic conversations, a curtain falls between lovers. For some, the reduction in communication is slight. For most, however, the curtain is heavy and dark. Thoreau spoke for modern man when he wrote over a hundred years ago, "The mass of men lead lives of quiet desperation." Alienation and secrets are of special concern in sexuality, which should be an intimate, sharing experience. Intimate, loving communication can break this curtain and personal isolation.

Sexuality has many functions in a relationship. It is a means of sharing pleasure, of reinforcing and deepening intimacy, and of reducing tension to help couples cope with the hassles of marriage and everyday life. An additional function is procreation, especially having a planned, wanted child.

Nearly everybody at some time in his or her life finds it difficult to verbally express love, caring, or even concern. Touching and nonverbal requests serve to bridge gaps and allow couples to connect. Both verbal and nonverbal communication is vital.

No matter what else you do with this book, then, we urge you to find or make ways to communicate your interest, caring, and desire for intimacy. Tell your partner what you appreciate and value about him or her. An intimate relationship is one of life's major satisfactions.

The exercises should be tried only after you and your partner have read and discussed them. What have you experienced and what do you want to experience? Talk about feelings of intimacy and caring as well as erotic scenarios and techniques. It takes effort to break through the natural hesitation you feel, but the personal and relational benefits can be immeasurable.

Be sure to tell your partner what you like and dislike. Many people want to talk about sexual odors (turn-ons and turn-offs) but cannot bring themselves to air that subject. Our culture has many sensitivities about hygiene so sexual partners deprive themselves of pleasurable experiences (or expose themselves to unpleasant experiences) for fear of mentioning sexual odors. Talk about what is important to you—fantasies, sounds, settings, smells, positions, temperature, amount of light. Feel free to make sexual requests. Breaking free of cultural restrictions helps your sexual relationship become open and satisfying.

Expressing Feelings

How can you express feelings? Each individual and couple develop their own style of expression. Here are suggestions and guidelines.

1. "I desire you." It can be validating to admit desire and energizing to feel desirable. The expression of desire reinforces your partner's sense of personal and sexual worth and promotes intimate communication. You can "desire" your partner in affectionate, sensual, playful, and erotic ways.

2. "You make me feel good." This is almost a definition of a good lover. It is important to tell your partner that he or she pleases you. Feeling good is not limited to sexual expression. It includes respect, trust, and emotional intimacy.

3. "I care about you." Expression of interest and concern is especially important in times of stress and trouble, but is always welcome, including during happy times. It is a fact of human behavior that *expressing* care increases the amount of genuine intimacy. Caring and sharing increase sexual desire.

Planning Exercises

After you complete the non-genital and genital pleasuring exercises, share what you have learned individually and as a couple. Then discuss what you want to try next. You might decide to focus on exercises to enhance your sexual relationship, exercises dealing with a specific sexual problem, or exercises which integrate intercourse with pleasuring. Proceed according to your needs rather than to the order of the book.

In subsequent exercises, we suggest following the approach of reading a chapter individually, discussing it as a couple, and choosing whether to proceed. Discuss how you will integrate intercourse with the exercises. We recommend that not every exercise end in intercourse. One possibility is to have intercourse at times other than when you are doing the exercises. Another is to complete an exercise and then go to intercourse if both are interested. Utilize the exercises so you get the most learning and enjoyment from each without putting pressure on yourself or your partner. Sexuality is about sharing pleasure, not proving anything or performing for your partner.

It is our hope that this book and these exercises will make you aware of and comfortable with a view of sexuality in which the pleasures of touching, intercourse, and afterplay flow in a natural, comfortable manner. Orgasm is the natural culmination of sexual arousal, not the ultimate goal which you have to achieve. We advocate an attitude toward sexuality that encompasses your whole body, not just your genitals, and considers affectionate, sensual, playful and erotic touching as valuable as intercourse. Communicate sexual needs and preferences in a sensitive, open manner.

There are chapters you might read without going through the exercises. Although you can benefit from just reading, we encourage you to experience the exercises so you can be comfortable with developing your couple sexual style. Psychological and sexual functioning is enhanced when the individual's attitudes, feelings, and behavior are congruent and reinforce each other. Reading the exercises helps modify attitudes. Doing the exercises (and thereby increasing comfort and skill) changes behavior. Being aware of reactions and giving and receiving feedback changes feelings. In these many and different ways we hope that you as a couple will grow in sexual awareness, comfort, pleasure, and satisfaction.

2

Information and Guidelines

How much do you really know about sexuality and sexual functioning? Many people believe they know all there is to know. Are you willing to take a test? Do not worry about performance anxiety—it will not be graded.

True-False Test

1. Sexual expression is purely natural, not a function of learning or communication.
2. Foreplay is for the woman; intercourse is for the man.
3. Once a couple establishes a good sexual relationship, they do not need to set aside time for intimacy.
4. If you love each other and communicate, everything will be fine sexually.
5. Sex and love are two sides of the same coin.
6. Technique is more important than intimacy in achieving sexual satisfaction.
7. Casual sex is more fun than intimate sex.
8. In a good relationship, each sexual experience is mutually satisfying.
9. Interest in sex decreases over the years and is lost by age sixty.

10. It is the man's role to initiate sex.
11. If one or both partners become aroused, intercourse must follow or there will be frustration.
12. Men and women are very different sexually; males are more sexually oriented.
13. Having "G" spot and multiple orgasms proves you are a sexually liberated woman.
14. Since men have few spontaneous erections after age fifty, they are less able to have intercourse.
15. When you lose sexual desire, the best remedy is to seek a new partner.
16. The most common female sexual problem is pain during intercourse.
17. The most common male sexual problem is lack of variety.
18. There is a significant relationship between the size of the man's penis and the woman's ability to reach orgasm.
19. Oral-genital sex is an exciting but perverse sexual behavior.
20. Simultaneous orgasms provide the most erotic pleasure.
21. Married people do not masturbate.
22. Using sexual fantasies during intercourse indicates dissatisfaction with your partner.
23. The woman has two kinds of orgasms—clitoral and vaginal.
24. Male-on-top is the most natural position for intercourse.
25. Viagra cures almost all erectile dysfunction.
26. People are doing much better sexually than the previous generation.

Add the number of *true's* you checked, and discover the number of sex myths you believe. For this was a sex-myth test—all the answers are false. Do not be surprised; the average number checked true is nine. Sexual myths are rampant in our culture, and they die hard.

We can all benefit from greater understanding of human sexuality. Knowledge is power. There has been a great deal of research and writing in the sexuality field during the past thirty years. Unfortunately, a whole new group of sophisticated, performance-oriented myths have replaced the old myths.

New Information—Positive Guidelines

We have more information about human sexuality than any culture in the history of the world. Yet there is no evidence that people are functioning better sexually or enjoying their sex lives more—contrary to the media myth that everyone is liberated and having great sex. We have gone from a sexually repressed, ignorant, and inhibited culture to a sex-saturated, performance-oriented, ambivalent, and confused sexual culture.

This book tries to provide up-to-date scientific information about sexuality and sexual functioning. The more information people have, the better they can choose how to integrate sexuality into their lives. Sexuality is your responsibility, not the responsibility of the culture, religion, schools, parents, or friends, although they can and do influence your sexual values and decisions. Sexuality is neither value-free nor governed by rules set in concrete. We attempt to provide guidelines for sexual awareness, functioning, and decision-making. Let us clearly state our value positions.

1. Sexuality is a good, healthy part of life, not bad or evil.
2. Sexuality is a positive, integral part of each individual's personality.
3. You are responsible for choosing how to express your sexuality. Sexuality can enhance your life and intimate relationship. It need not be a cause of anxiety, guilt, or problems.
4. A healthy sexual relationship is based on respect, trust, and intimacy.
5. An intimate relationship is the most secure and satisfying way to express sexuality.

Let us examine self-defeating myths and replace them with accurate information and attitudes which increase awareness and enhance sexual functioning.

1. Sexual Expression Is Both Natural and Learned

You are a sexual person from the day you are born until the day you die. For both women and men, sexual arousal occurs as a natural physiological function during the sleep cycle. The potential for sexual response is natural for all people.

Attitudes, behavior, and feelings develop as part of a complex process of sexual socialization and experiences. Sexual learning occurs throughout life; negative learnings and experiences can be overcome.

2. Pleasuring and Intercourse Are Mutual Activities

Artificial rigid roles for men and women inhibit sexual satisfaction. The foreplay/pleasuring period can be involving and enjoyable for the man as well as the woman. Rather than the man "doing" the woman so she is aroused enough for intercourse, both can enjoy the give-and-take pleasuring experience. Intercourse, too, is a mutual activity which can be as enjoyable and arousing for the woman as for the man. The best aphrodisiac is an involved, aroused partner. The "give to get" guideline means giving your partner pleasure gives you pleasure.

3. A Satisfying Sexual Relationship Needs Continual Time and Nurturing

You cannot take your sexual relationship for granted. Establishing a satisfying sexual relationship requires communication, caring, and sharing. You need to devote time and psychological energy to nurture and maintain a vital sexual relationship. Setting aside couple time (not all of which involves sexual activity) is the chief guideline for maintaining an intimate relationship. Sex can become routine and stagnant, especially when done late at night with little variety, communication, or experimentation. If you value sexuality, invest time, emotion, and energy into nurturing your intimate relationship.

4. Love and Communication Are Not Enough

There is a romantic myth that if you are in love and communicate, sex always works well. If the man is an early ejaculator or the woman has vaginismus (spasming of the vaginal opening), all the love and communication in the world will not solve the problem. Increasing sexual comfort and learning specific sexual skills are necessary. There are a number of loving couples who communicate feelings and work together in parenting, yet they are unable to transfer this caring and sharing to sexual functioning. Communication is necessary, but not sufficient. To overcome sexual problems, you need to learn and practice sexual communication and sexual skills.

5. Sex and Love Are Not the Same

The most human and satisfying relationships integrate intimacy and sexuality. Sex and love, however, are not the same. This myth has done immeasurable harm. When we speak of love, we do not mean the romantic high which comes intensely but fleetingly early in a relationship. Love evolves into a mature intimacy whereby you respect, trust, and care about each other. Sex is not limited to the initial excitement that comes with knowing you are attracted to and excited by a new person. Sexual function involves not only experiencing desire, arousal, and orgasm but also feeling emotionally satisfied and bonded. You can be sexually functional with people you do not even like, and can love someone but still have a chronic sexual problem. Sex and love are different. The most secure relationship integrates a loving intimacy with sexual satisfaction.

6. Technique vs. Intimacy

Many people dislike sex books because they emphasize technique (many do read like sophisticated sexual cookbooks) rather than emotional intimacy. We attempt to integrate sexual comfort and skills with emotional expression and with the trust and caring of an intimate relationship. For full sexual awareness, both sexual skills and emotional intimacy are crucial.

7. Casual Sex vs. Intimate Sex

Although an intimate sexual relationship is a valued goal, most people have experienced casual sexual relationships, especially in their teenage and young adult years. There is an excitement and illicitness in casual sex that are difficult to replicate in a marital relationship. An intimate relationship involves caring, trust, and security (including freedom from fears of STDs and HIV/AIDS and from coercion), which are not possible in casual sexual encounters.

8. Variability in Sexual Relationships

Unrealistic expectations place a heavy burden on a sexual relationship. No matter how great the intimacy or how inventive the technique, not every sexual encounter can be "dynamite." In fact, couples with a healthy sexual relationship report that in only 40 to 50 percent of their sexual encounters do they find desire, arousal, orgasm and satisfaction equal. In 5 to 15 percent of sexual interactions the sex will be mediocre, unsatisfying, or unsuccessful—the kind where in the middle one says, "I hope you're enjoying this," and the partner responds, "No, I'm doing this for you." Couples who can laugh or shrug this off and try again the next day when they are receptive and responsive will maintain satisfying sex. We are not sexual machines who perform perfectly on demand. If all sex were like a five-course steak-and-lobster dinner with the finest wine, it would become routine and dull. Variability and flexibility are a normal aspect of sexual expression. The expectation that both partners should be equally involved, orgasmic, and satisfied every time is unrealistic.

9. People Are Sexual at Sixty and Beyond

Some of the cruelest myths involve sex and aging. If you are in good health, have an interested partner, and a positive attitude toward sexuality, you can enjoy sex into your sixties, seventies, and beyond. Physiological changes with aging are gradual rather than dramatic and alter sexual functioning rather than stop it. The more you understand

and accept normal bodily changes, the easier it is to integrate these into your sexual relationship. The major advantage of sex after sixty is you spend more time in sensual and sexual pleasuring since lubrication in women and erection in men take longer. Emotional intimacy, non-demand pleasuring and erotic stimulation reach their greatest fruition as a couple ages.

10. Both Can Initiate; Both Can Say No

Sexual myths and bad habits develop during the dating period. One of the most harmful is that it is the man's role to initiate and there is something wrong with the woman who wants and initiates sex. Sex is a shared pleasure; each person has the right to initiate and to say no. Men have more trouble learning to say no than women have learning to make clear, direct sexual initiations and requests. He feels "to be a real man, he should be able to have sex at any time and in any place." His being comfortable saying no when he does not want intercourse allows the woman to be freer in her initiations and allows both to enjoy a range of sensual and erotic activities.

11. Not All Touching Has to Proceed to Intercourse

Couples can be comfortable touching whether they are clothed or nude, whether they are inside or outside the bedroom, for they are not inhibited by the fear that if one becomes aroused and the other does not desire intercourse, frustration and an argument will follow. Pleasure and arousal are valuable in themselves, not just as a prelude to intercourse. Touching is a way to connect for affection, to express sensuality, or to share eroticism. People who avoid touch unless they want intercourse cheat themselves and their relationship. Touching is integral to an intimate relationship. Couples who touch in a variety of situations have more frequent intercourse because they share connection and pleasure, pleasure which may be enjoyed for itself or proceed to intercourse.

12. Men and Women Are More Alike Sexually Than Different

The major theme of the double standard was that men are interested in sex and that women are interested in the relationship and merely submit to sex. Sex researchers, however, find that the same physiological processes underlie male and female sexuality; there are many more similarities than differences. Women have the potential to be multi-orgasmic, so if you just used the criterion of orgasm, you could argue that women are more sexual. These arguments fuel competitiveness and misunderstanding. An empowering concept is that both men and women value intimacy, pleasuring and eroticism. The most satisfied couples integrate emotional and sexual expression.

13. The Tyranny of Female Orgasm

Women now experience the same performance pressure which has so plagued men. The pressure to prove she is liberated by having multiple orgasms or identifying her "G" spot and having the perfect orgasm is scientifically wrong and psychologically self-defeating. Female orgasm (like male orgasm) is the natural culmination of sexual involvement, erotic stimulation, increasing arousal, and letting go. Women have different patterns and preferences for being orgasmic. No two people are exactly the same sexually. Arbitrarily judging an orgasm as "right," "mature," or "liberated" is self-negating. A healthy attitude emphasizes sharing sexual pleasure, not viewing sex as a performance. Sex is about pleasuring, not proving something to yourself or your partner.

14. Spontaneous Erections and Intercourse

For males under twenty-five, spontaneous erections are the rule. As a man ages, the frequency and intensity of spontaneous erections gradually decline, most noticeably in the forties and fifties. Instead of erection being easy, automatic, and autonomous, arousal is a result of partner stimulation and the give and take of pleasuring. Arousal and erection become a function of intimate, interactive sexuality. For the man over fifty, it takes longer to get an erection and requires direct penile stimulation. The good news is that sexuality becomes increasingly more an involved, shared cooperative activity as partners age. Couples can continue to enjoy erections and intercourse into their sixties, seventies, and beyond. Lack of spontaneous erection does not mean lack of sexual desire or the ability to enjoy arousal, erection, and intercourse.

15. Regaining Sexual Desire

Inhibited sexual desire is the most common sexual dysfunction at the beginning of this century. There are a number of factors which can inhibit desire including anger, depression, abuse of alcohol or drugs, disappointment or frustration with the partner, chronic illness, side effects of medications, an arousal or orgasm dysfunction, lack of couple time. Sexual problems devitalize an intimate relationship. The majority of couples, especially those in a committed relationship, can resolve sexual difficulties. Once inhibitions and blocks in sexual communication are identified and addressed, sexual desire can be revitalized.

16. Common Female Sexual Problems

Although a significant number of women experience painful intercourse on occasion (caused by fatigue, low arousal, anger, lack of lubrication, anxiety, and poor technique), this is usually not a chronic problem. Spending time on pleasuring, the woman guiding penile intromission, using a lubricant, or switching intercourse positions usually alleviates the pain. The most common female sexual problems are inhibited sexual desire, lack of arousal, orgasmic dysfunction, and dissatisfaction with couple intimacy.

17. Common Male Sexual Problems

Men tend to brag about and exaggerate their sexual exploits and joke about never having enough sex. In reality, about 50 percent of men have a sexual dysfunction or dissatisfaction, which they are loath to admit even to their partner. Men are sexual people, not sexual machines. The most common male sexual problems are early ejaculation, erectile dysfunction, inhibited sexual desire, and ejaculatory inhibition (difficulty reaching orgasm).

18. The Myth of Penis Size

Many men—indeed, 75 percent—worry their penis is smaller than average. Statistically, that is absurd, but it is even more misdirected from a psychological viewpoint. There are a wide range of penis sizes in the flaccid state. This evens out when the penis becomes erect (larger penises grow in circumference but less so in length, and smaller penises grow in length and circumference), so in the erect state there are minimal size differences. The difference that exists does not matter since the vagina is an adaptable organ which adjusts to the penis inserted. The major nerve endings are in the outer third of the vagina, so larger does not mean better. Males spend hours worrying about penis size and feeling self-conscious about something which is a myth and has nothing to do with male or female sexual satisfaction.

19. Oral-genital Sexuality

A major change in sexual behavior over the past twenty years is the growing popularity of oral-genital sex, both fellatio and cunnilingus. Couples who utilize oral-genital pleasuring techniques report higher levels of satisfaction. Fellatio and cunnilingus do not replace intercourse; they are complementary sexual activities. Variety, experimentation, and communication enhance sexual satisfaction. Oral-genital sex is a special turn-on, which facilitates arousal and satisfaction.

20. Simultaneous Orgasm:
A Performance Myth

Orgasm is a three- to ten-second experience for men and women. Sex manuals herald simultaneous orgasm as the ultimate sexual experience. Trying to reach this rigid performance goal has frustrated untold numbers of couples. Orchestrating sexual arousal so that both people reach their emotional and physical climax at exactly the same time is more a task for engineers than lovers. Some couples enjoy reaching orgasm at the same time, although few report it to be the overwhelming experience promised by the books. Others report simultaneous orgasm as pleasant, but are disappointed by the lack of intensity. We suggest a less goal-oriented approach to sexuality—accept and enjoy an orgasm in whatever sequence you experience it.

21. Married People Masturbate

Masturbation is a normal, healthy sexual behavior at fifteen, thirty-five, or sixty-five, whether you are single, divorced, or married. The majority of both married men and woman masturbate on occasion. There are many reasons to masturbate: when you are physically separated from your spouse, when you want to enjoy your sexual responsiveness and fantasies, when you feel sexual but your partner does not. Masturbation can serve negative purposes, such as avoiding partner sex, indulging in an obsessive fantasy, or compulsively using Internet sex, but any sexual behavior can be misused. Masturbation is not a regressive, adolescent behavior. It is a normal, positive sexual expression for both women and men that occurs throughout life.

22. The Positive Functions of Sexual Fantasy

Both men and women utilize sexual fantasies. Fantasies can elicit sexual desire and serve as a bridge to arousal, a form of multiple stimulation, or a rehearsal for partner sex. A large majority of both men and women use sexual fantasies, at least occasionally, during partner sex. Fantasies seldom involve the partner. What makes fantasies erotic is that they are illicit and socially unacceptable. Does that mean that the sex you fantasize is the sex you really want? Not at all. People fantasize about being sexually humiliated or raped; this can make for an arousing fantasy but would be a traumatic sexual experience. Fantasies are in a different realm than sexual behavior. People utilize them to intensify their pleasure during partner sex.

23. The Clitoral vs. Vaginal Orgasm Myth

Physiologically, an orgasm is an orgasm whether it occurs during masturbation, cunnilingus, intercourse, vibrator stimulation, or manual stimulation. Depending on the woman's attitudes, expectations, preferences, and experiences, her psychological satisfaction will vary. The old view of "mature vs. immature" orgasms or "more feminine vs. less feminine" orgasmic response simply is not true. The clitoral area has the most sexual nerve endings and the clitoris is indirectly stimulated by a number of arousal techniques, including intercourse. The woman's (and her partner's) accepting her pattern of orgasm is the most psychologically enhancing way to deal with myths and demands concerning female orgasm.

24. Intercourse Variations

Male-on-top intercourse is the most commonly used in our culture because it is the easiest position for the man to guide intromission and to prevent the penis from slipping out of the vagina. It is a fine intercourse position and has advantages for both men and women. However, there is nothing "natural," "superior," or "the right way" about it. In some cultures, man-on-top is rarely used. Most couples enjoy experimenting with other intercourse positions such as woman-on-top, side-by-side, rear entry, standing, and kneeling. Couples develop their unique style of being sexual, which includes preferred variations of intercourse positions.

25. Integrating Viagra into the Couple Lovemaking Style

The trend of medicalizing male sexuality (as well as female sexuality) with Viagra-type drugs and testosterone enhancement is misguided and ultimately self-defeating. Viagra can be a helpful drug and in the coming years a new generation of pro-sexual drugs, creams and patches will be introduced. However, unless these are integrated with a couple's intimacy, pleasuring and eroticism, they will not help either the individual or the couple in the long run. Medical intervention works best as a supplemental resource to enhance your couple sexual style.

26. Making Sexuality a Positive, Integral Part of the Relationship

The myth that people are doing much better sexually than their parents' generation is one myth we wish were true. Sexuality is discussed more openly, and there is greater scientific knowledge. People are having intercourse at an earlier age. There is an increase in sexual experimentation, STDs, AIDS, and extramarital affairs. Is there an increase in sexual awareness, pleasure, and intimacy? Has the increase in sexual quantity led to an increase in sexual quality and satisfaction? It has for some people, but not for the majority. The number of "casualties of the sexual revolution" through sexual trauma, STDs, AIDS, and failed relationships continues to grow. Our goal is to increase sexual awareness, enhance sexual intimacy, and make sexuality a positive, integral part of your life and intimate relationship.

Sexual Guidelines

The following chapters present concepts and exercises to increase your awareness, comfort, pleasure, and satisfaction. Freeing yourself from self-defeating attitudes and myths is an important step. Adopting sexual attitudes, behavior, and feelings that promote and enhance your sexuality and intimate relationship is the focus of this book.

II

Sexual Comfort and Pleasure

3

Sensuality: Non-Genital Pleasuring

Many couples find that their sexual life has become mechanical and unsatisfying. Their sexual expression has gotten so narrowly focused on intercourse with the goal of orgasm that they think back to their first sexual experiences and remember with fondness feelings of excitement, playfulness, spontaneity, and seductive touching. They wonder what they have lost and how it happened. Intercourse and orgasm have overshadowed the joys of pleasurable touching, sensual feelings, and broad-based sexuality. Playfulness and enjoyment have been replaced by a pattern in which all touching leads to intercourse. Fun and spontaneity have disappeared and been replaced by a rigid goal orientation, which pressures the couple to make each sex experience perfect.

The focus of this chapter is reorienting yourselves toward pleasurable, sensual feelings. The emphasis will be on discovering, in a relaxed, non–goal-oriented manner, the sensual pleasure you can derive from touching and being touched. It allows you to discover or rediscover the style of touching, stroking, and caressing which feels comfortable and pleasurable. Couples develop assumptions (often based on misperceptions), fall into ruts, and feel awkward asking for a different type of touching. These exercises are designed to increase comfort with touching, discovering, and sharing with as little performance demand or goal-orientation as possible.

The exercises are suggestions and flexible guidelines rather than rigid rules. Their purpose is to explore and experience. They are designed to facilitate feeling comfortable as a sensual and sexual couple, not prove anything to yourself or your partner. They are about intimate feelings and sensuality, not a sexual performance. If you accept yourself as a sensual being, you will be better able to focus on your partner and appreciate his/her feelings, needs, and sensitivities.

Time and privacy are crucial. It is important not to be distracted by factors such as the phone ringing, people coming over, or children walking in. Plan a time, between half an hour and an hour and a half, when you will not be disturbed—when the children are asleep, with a baby-sitter, or at friends' houses.

Lock the bedroom door (if you do not have a lock make the investment and buy one; it will pay sexual dividends). Take the phone off the hook or put the answering machine on. Each exercise can take from thirty to ninety minutes, depending on your feelings and preferences. You are encouraged to proceed in a gradual, step-by-step fashion, so as to become comfortable with one experience before moving on to the next. It is important to feel comfortable and receptive so you can explore, discover, and enjoy sensual feelings.

Begin the exercise by bathing or showering together. We recommend this for two reasons: first, it serves to relax you and enhance comfortable feelings about your body; second, proper care and cleanliness are important in enhancing sensual feelings.

At this point we should mention the subject of "no." Suppose one person suggests a sensual or sexual activity and the other is not interested. The partner who is denied may feel rejected and avoid further contact if his initiation is met with a no. Rather than simply saying no, propose an alternative you would be receptive to. This principle applies to all sexual activity, and cannot be overemphasized. Refrain from saying no; suggest sensual or sexual alternatives or another time to be together. You might say, "No, I don't want to have intercourse now, but I would like to have my back rubbed or to hold hands and talk." Or: "I don't want a massage, but I would like to lie and hold." This keeps the dialogue open. It allows the partner to say that although one activity does not appeal, something else does. It affirms an interest in sensual or sexual contact and in maintaining an intimate connection.

Intimate communication lies at the heart of a satisfying sexual experience. If the partner initiates an activity with caring and consideration, and the person responds by expressing her feelings clearly and openly, this reinforces intimacy.

Many people find appearance important. Often individuals fall into the trap of not being aware of their appearance, especially when just with their partner. They fail to fix their hair, do not wear fresh clothing or brush their teeth, or maintain a healthy weight. Lack of care can detract from sexual attractiveness. For some, the trap is always dressing formally, being so fastidious that they lose their natural attractiveness. Another trap is the requisite that one feel perfect and beautiful for sex, which is likely to result in the avoidance of sex. Individuals vary in what they find attractive and sensual, so it is important to be aware of your desires and feelings and learn your partner's preferences. Remember, the essence of sexuality is two comfortable, involved people giving and receiving pleasure-oriented touching.

Joan and Andy

Joan and Andy consulted Barry after seven years of marriage. It was Joan's first marriage and Andy's second. They were part of the "liberation" movement of the 1960s and thought of themselves as sexually free and sophisticated. Their sexual relationship was excellent while living together and for the first ten months after marriage, but it became increasingly unsatisfying and had fallen off precipitously in the past three years. Andy and Joan had been in couple therapy and couple group therapy. They had explored a number of relationship issues, including financial problems, dealing with in-laws, power struggles, adolescent stepchildren, and avoidance of intimacy. Some issues were successfully dealt with; others remained problematic.

Joan and Andy continued to search for the nonsexual causes of their sexual problem—they could not imagine how two such sexually sophisticated and experienced people could have a sexual dysfunction. When Barry confronted their pattern of minimal touching, which might lead either to a "dynamite" sexual intercourse or to a bitter, frustrating argument, they were taken aback. When given the prescription for non-genital pleasuring exercises, they were resistant. Andy and Joan saw non-genital stimulation as an excercise for people who were sexually anxious and inhibited, not for them. While it is true that these exercises are designed to increase comfort with nudity, touching, and initiating for couples who are anxious and inhibited, they also provide an experience most couples (including you) can benefit from. If you ignore non-demand sensuous experiences, it is hard to have a satisfying sexual relationship. Sensuality is the basis of sexual response and a crucial ingredient in maintaining a satisfying intimate relationship.

Andy and Joan found the exercises of great benefit. They reawakened forgotten pleasurable feelings of being caressed and touched for their own sake. Joan and Andy rediscovered a playful, comfortable manner of being with each other. A second, and unexpected, effect was to elicit specific problems in their manner of sexual expression. Under the thin guise of liberation, there were serious difficulties in stating feelings, acknowledging intimacy, and being open to the needs and requests of the partner. They learned that by not retreating into anger, they could continue to share sensuality and feel safe and trusting, which increased intimacy.

As you prepare to engage in the exercises, be aware of what you want to learn and experience with non–goal-oriented, non-demand pleasuring. Give yourself permission to explore, feel, and share.

First Set of Exercises: Exploration

Before beginning, sit and talk for ten or fifteen minutes, perhaps over a cup of coffee or one glass of wine. Contrary to popular mythology, alcohol is a central nervous system depressant that interferes with arousal (although it can temporarily facilitate desire). Recall a particular experience when you felt close and intimate. Express this feeling.

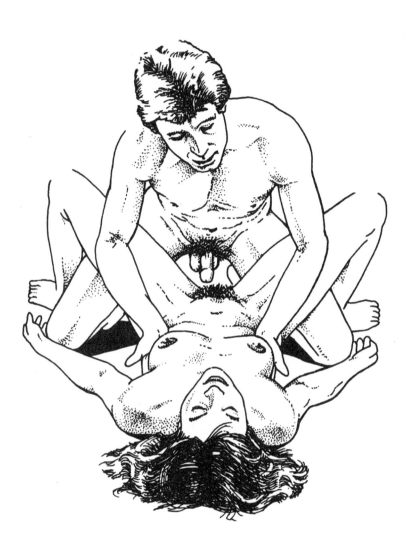

Non-genital pleasuring: male as pleasure-giver; female as recipient.

Put your hands palms-down on the table. Ask your partner to do the same, and allow your hands to be caressed. Notice the differences in size and texture. Much can be communicated by hands touching.

If you shower as a prelude to pleasuring, experiment with different types of spray or temperature; if bathing, try a new bath oil or soap. This can increase awareness of sensual stimuli. Start by soaping your partner's back, caressing as you do so. Trace the muscles and contours; gently rub and massage. Ask your partner to face you. Soap the front of the neck and chest, but go around the breasts. Touch especially the hollows of the neck and the soft area below the ribs and navel. Move downward to the hips, bypassing the genital area. Wash your own genitals. Soap your partner's legs while telling him or her how it feels. Let your partner soap you. Be aware of what feels particularly sensuous.

When you have finished, dry each other, except for genitals. Take your time; being slow and tender is also important here. Stand still for a moment and take a good look at your partner. See your partner as a new person. Notice one or two things you find particularly attractive and share them. Walk toward each other, hands extended and hold your partner's hands. Slide your partner's arms around your waist; enjoy the closeness. Feel and share as you begin a new warmth, closeness, and intimacy.

Proceed to your bedroom and feel natural being nude. If you do not feel comfortable walking through the house nude, put on a robe or towel, but leave it when you reach the bedroom. Pleasuring is best done in the nude. Later, you can vary the amount of clothing (which can be tantalizing), but first learn to be comfortable with your own and your partner's nudity. The room should be at a comfortable, warm temperature with a moderate amount of light. If you prefer, partially darken the room, only be sure you can see your partner's body. If you like, put your favorite music on the radio or CD and/or burn a candle with a pleasant fragrance.

Designate one partner the pleasure-giver and the other pleasure-recipient. Typically, you will switch roles during the exercise, though some prefer to do one session as the giver and the next as receiver. Be sure each partner has an opportunity to do both, since a mutually satisfying relationship requires both being comfortable receiving and giving. Interestingly, many people (especially males) find it harder to receive than to give. Neither role carries connotations of dominance or submission, of femininity or masculinity.

The recipient has three tasks. The first is to be passive and receive pleasure. The second is to keep your eyes closed throughout the exercise so as to be able to concentrate on feelings and sensations. The third task is to be aware of what parts of your body and what types of touch are sensuous.

Let the male begin as giver. He should view his partner in a new way and feel comfortable giving her a wide variety of touch and body stimulation. Rather than trying to second-guess her, he should touch for himself—engage in stimulation he enjoys giving. The recipient is lying on her stomach, feeling as receptive, relaxed, and comfortable as possible. You can look at and touch your partner from the top of her head to the bottoms of her feet. This exercise focuses on the back of her body; the second exercise on the front. Throughout this exercise, the emphasis is on communication by touch rather than words, so both should refrain from talking or joking. Talking distracts from focusing on sensations and feelings. Begin by massaging her shoulders. Gently massage, being careful not to squeeze the upper neck muscles. Rub tenderly with the entire hand, moving slowly down the back and sides; try to avoid sudden movements. Be aware of what is appealing that you might not have noticed before—freckles, tiny scars, muscle indentations. When you reach her waist, place your thumbs together, spread your fingers, and press and knead gently as you caress her sides and lower back. Move to the head, and either give a scalp massage or gently run your fingers through her hair. Return to the back, but this time press vigorously and give a back rub. You might like to run your fingers over your partner's back in a playful, disorganized manner. You could trace special features of her back with your fingertips.

The task of the giver is to provide the recipient with a variety of experiences so she can increase awareness of sensual feelings. The giver

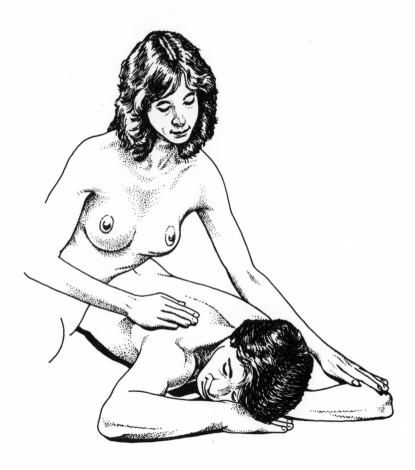

Non-genital pleasuring: female as pleasure-giver; male as recipient.

can enjoy trying various types of touching and experience her body in a new way. The emphasis is on exploring rather than working to arouse the partner or prove yourself sexually. Feel comfortable; enjoy it. These exercises are guidelines, not hard and fast rules to follow like a cookbook. Feel free to be creative, playful, and innovative.

Hold your partner's feet and caress them. Notice the length of the toes, the texture of the nails. Place your palm so it covers the arch, and curl your fingers over the top of the foot. Notice the heel as you rub the palm of your hand against it. Outline the division between the top and bottom of her foot with your fingertips. Holding one foot, caress the top with your fingers and trace the valleys between the toes. Gently massage the foot up to the ankle. Moving up the same leg, hold the ankle in one hand while exploring it with the other hand. Gently and slowly move up the calf, caressing and massaging to help your partner relax even more. Pay attention to rubbing the soft area behind the knee. Examine and explore her thigh; look for little places you have not touched before. Move to the buttocks and massage both simultaneously. Some people feel negative about this area because of the association with defecation. The buttocks and anal area can be one of the most sensuous parts of the body; they comprise an erogenous zone with a multitude of nerve endings. Touch in a manner that is enjoyable and sensuous.

When you have provided a non-demand sensuous exploration, switch giver and recipient roles and repeat the pleasuring experience. There can be large differences in the time spent, ranging between fifteen to seventy-five minutes per person. The giver can explore and touch in his or her own way. This is not a "tit for tat" game. The focus is on exploring, enjoying, touching, learning, comfort, and sensuality. The key concepts are *slow, tender, rhythmic, caring.*

After this exercise, sit over a drink or cup of coffee, discuss the experience, and share feelings. Because talking tends to isolate you from bodily feelings, it is best to do the exercise in silence. Afterward, we encourage sharing and processing feelings and reactions in a direct, open manner. We suggest you do this clothed over the kitchen table or on a walk. Processing a sexual experience while nude in bed is too vulnerable, especially when dealing with sensitive or difficult feed-back. First share positive feelings and then say what was problematic. Try to maintain a 5 to 1 positive–negative ratio. Rather than seeing the negative as blame or a put-down, view it as constructive with requests and suggestions of what to try next time.

Second Set of Exercises: Guiding

Begin by taking a bath or shower. Make it more relaxed, comfortable, and sensuous than the first time. Dry your partner, commenting and sharing as you do. The female begins as giver so she can become comfortable with initiating, while the male can become comfortable with being passive and accepting pleasure.

In this excercise the male keeps his eyes open and guides his part-ner's hands to sensuous, pleasurable areas of his back. He is free to use touch or words to guide and make requests.

The receiver should find at least two areas on the back of his body that are particularly sensuous and let the giver know so that she can be fully aware of his preferences. The giver can use kissing and lick-ing. This includes kissing the back of her partner's neck, running her tongue from the top to the bottom of his spinal cord, blowing in the ear and flicking her tongue in and out, and taking gentle "love bites" on his legs. Different people like different things. Partners do not know what each likes until they try. This is not a test; there are no right or wrong responses. Explore and enjoy.

When the giver feels ready, she can help her partner turn over on his back. The receiver now keeps his eyes closed, relaxes, and assumes a passive, receptive attitude. Males are not used to the passive role, but it is important to experience being passive and receptive to learn what sensual feelings they are most responsive to. The giver can visually examine the front of the partner's body and notice what parts are particularly attractive.

Then cover his hand with yours. Notice differences in size and texture. Gently massage the fingers, then run your fingertips along the palm. Slide your fingers down his hand and look for things you have not noticed before. Trace the knuckles and small lines on his fingers. Gently kiss the soft inner palm of each hand. Caress your partner's forearms, one at a time. Notice the softness of the skin on the inner side of the arm. Trace the elbow with your fingers. Placing your thumb in the bend, grasp the forearm and slide your hand down to the wrist. Caress both arms in their entirety.

Gently explore his face. Notice the signs of relaxation and comfort; be aware of the difference between these expressions and the tension you observe in other situations. To enhance feelings of relaxation and sensuousness, gently massage his forehead. Move from his cheeks to the chin, and with your fingertips outline favorite facial features. You might tenderly kiss your partner's closed eyes. In fact, you might want to kiss all the parts of his face.

You can massage around his nipples and see if touching them feels sensuous. Many males find this sensual, but inhibit their natural response because they think men are not supposed to feel good there. When you are exploring the chest, use smooth, tender strokes and cover the sides as well. Move up to the armpit and run your hands over it. Notice the feel of his hair on your hands. How does it feel to touch your partner's navel? Run your hands sideways around his stomach. Be aware of how stomach muscles react to your touch. Avoid the genital area, but do explore sensuous touch around the inner thighs.

It may happen at this point or elsewhere in the exercises you feel sexual arousal. The male may get an erection and the female may vaginally lubricate. Accept this as a natural, healthy, sexual response. If it does not happen, that is fine too; the purpose is to explore, learn, and enjoy sensuality. Non-genital pleasuring is a comfortable experience without pressure for sexual arousal.

Explore the front of his legs and feet. In ending this exercise, visually reexamine the front of your partner's body and caress the two or three areas you find most attractive. Remember, there are no right or wrong areas. Perceptions of attractiveness vary; you might especially like his eyes, neck, chest, inner thighs—touch what is appealing to you.

Switch giver-and-recipient roles, and repeat the touching sequence. During this exercise, the male as giver refrains from touching or caressing his partner's breasts. Each person does touching and pleasuring differently, which is as it should be since you are learning to be comfortable with your personal style of giving and receiving pleasure. Afterward, spend time discussing differences between your style and your partner's. How can you utilize these differences to make your sensual and sexual relationship more satisfying?

Third Set of Exercises: Mutuality

Sit across from each other, separated by a table. Make sure it is narrow enough so you can easily reach your partner's hands and face.

Put your hands palm-down on the table. Ask your partner to do the same and caress his hands. Cover your partner's hands with yours. Grasp gently and lift them from the table. Slide your hands underneath so they support your partner's. Releasing one hand, cover the other so it is enclosed within yours. Lift the hand to your face and rub the back on your cheeks, one then the other. Make eye contact as you do this. Repeat with your eyes closed.

Pick up both hands and place them on your face so they enclose it, from your cheeks to your chin. Close your eyes and slowly move your face from side to side. Holding the wrists, bend your neck forward, inclining your face toward your chest, and move his hands to the sides of your neck. Then raise your face, bring the hands together under the chin, and separate them so they slide up your face; stop when the fingertips reach your eyes. Gently kiss the soft inner palm of each hand. Make eye contact and communicate how you feel about the closeness.

Placing hands on the table, imagine you will never be allowed to touch again. How would you approach these hands if that were true—touch, squeeze, kiss them as if it were the last time. Share feelings about this experience and verbalize your sense of caring.

You can go directly to the touching exercises, or if you prefer, start with a shower or bath. The focus will be on guiding and teaching your partner what feels sensuous on the front of your body. Allow this to be a mutual give-and-take experience, moving away from the structured roles of giver and recipient. Keep eyes open so you can communicate feelings through eye contact. Most of the guiding will be nonverbal, using your hand over your partner's to show what kind of touch and where on your body the feelings are particularly good. To enhance the experience, we suggest using a lotion while massaging. People experiment with several varieties, including wild lemon lotion, aloe vera, abalone lotion, and baby oil. It can be fun to go shopping together and choose one or two lotions you would like to try. It is important to have the lotion readily available so you do not have to stop caressing to get it. If possible, heat the lotion. Cold lotion poured on bare skin can shock anyone out of a sensuous mood. If the lotion is not heated, leave one hand on your partner's body and pour the lotion onto the back of that hand. When it is warm, rub it on your partner's body.

Be aware of your partner's breathing. Find the rhythm of the breathing and follow it with the caressing motions of your hands. Be especially aware of the response to kissing or running your tongue over your partner's body. Mutually explore and share.

In ending this experience, lie with the male's chest against the woman's back, bodies touching, with his arms gently around her waist. Talk and share feelings. Then lie quietly until sleep overtakes you.

Fourth Set of Exercises: Sharing

Begin by discussing what degree of cleanliness is comfortable for you. Allow yourselves increasing amounts of mutuality, spontaneity, and playfulness. Both people can initiate touching and caressing, which will transfer into a mutually satisfying foreplay/pleasuring pattern. Let the touching and pleasuring remain non-genital. We suggest using a different lotion so awareness of various smells and sensuous feelings will be enhanced.

Try not to miss an opportunity to share honestly. Express feelings and make requests. Communicate your thoughts in new and different words. Express your desire for each other. Your body is learning to give and receive tenderness and warmth; your words can convey these new feelings. Let your partner know how special a person she or he truly is.

Try a different position. The woman can lie on her stomach, with the man lying on his side, facing her, and touching her entire body, his upper leg bent at the knee so his leg rests across her legs. Slowly and gently he can caress her back from the neck to the waist. He can gently move his leg up and down her legs, feeling her skin with the inside of his thigh and calf, while exploring and touching with the instep of his foot. Talk while touching. Tell her how you are feeling emotionally and physically. Ask how she is feeling, what she likes, and how you can please her.

Switch to a different position, perhaps kneeling and facing each other or lying across from each other. Exchange gentle, tender, mutual caresses. Enjoy simultaneously giving and receiving pleasure. Allow this to be a mutual sensuous, sharing experience, which can be repeated for itself or at a later time as part of pleasuring and lead to erotic stimulation, arousal, and intercourse.

Closing Thoughts

We hope you are aware and accepting of your body's natural responses to non-genital touch and the pleasures of sensuality. Couples can fall into a trap where the only touching they do is genital and leads to intercourse. We hope you have learned to appreciate feelings of sensuality and non-genital touch, are aware what kinds of non-genital touch are most enjoyable, and what parts of your body are responsive. Share this verbally and nonverbally, communicating in a direct, comfortable way.

With a basic foundation of acceptance of touch and an emphasis on slow, tender, warm, intimate sharing, you can progress to become a sexually expressive couple.

4

Genital Pleasuring

Through the non-genital exercises, you have become comfortable with your natural bodily feelings and with sharing sensuality. You've relearned the enjoyment of non-demand touching without worrying about the pressures of goal-oriented sexual performance. Now that the base of slow, gentle, caring, rhythmic touching has been established, you can build upon it by adding genital touch. Experience a natural, integrated approach to being a sensual and sexual couple. During these exercises, do not fall into the trap of having all interactions become genitally oriented, aimed toward arousal and orgasm. Instead, genital touching is preceded by and integrated with non-genital. They complement each other.

Continue to explore and enjoy giving and receiving pleasure. The *goal* of sexual intercourse is not appropriate at this point because it raises performance anxiety and distracts from the pleasure and arousal experience. The emphasis is on non-demand pleasuring, integrating non-genital with genital touching and sensual with sexual feelings.

Ruth and Kyle

Ruth and Kyle were an affectionate couple who felt good about their marriage. People thought of them as a "golden couple." Women friends would gossip, saying they wished their husbands were as affectionate

and caring as Kyle. Ruth and Kyle, however, had an embarrassing secret; their sexual relationship was nonexistent. Like one in five married couples they had intercourse less than ten times a year. They were
a couple who did well with affection, communication, and emotional
intimacy, but not with sensual or sexual encounters.

Barry assured Ruth and Kyle they had an excellent prognosis for
overcoming the problem since a committed couple who communicate
feelings and have a solid intimate relationship are the ideal sex therapy candidates. Their history revealed that sexual intercourse was a
major problem. Ruth was poorly lubricated and Kyle initiated quickly
and awkwardly. He ejaculated rapidly, which was fine with Ruth since
she did not derive pleasure from intercourse.

They had skipped a major step in the sexual process—the pleasure
and arousal which comes from genital touching and stimulation. Sexual stimulation was a perfunctory touch on the breasts and vagina, two
or three caresses, one or two hand strokes of the penis, and then on
to intercourse. A prohibition on intercourse was imposed in order to
give them the space and freedom to explore a variety of non-genital
and genital pleasuring techniques.

The first week of exercises brought a dramatic change as Ruth and
Kyle engaged in non-genital touching and discovered the joys of shared
sensuality. They particularly enjoyed showering together and engaging
in whole body massage. They felt more open and comfortable with nudity than they had in the past eight years.

The second week involved genital touch and exploration with a
ban on orgasm. The ban was lifted the third week with the guideline
that they could allow arousal to culminate naturally in orgasm if they
wished, but should not feel a demand or pressure to do so. Some couples enjoy being orgasmic with manual, oral, or rubbing stimulation;
others do not. Kyle and Ruth had never tried it. The process was a real
eye-opener; they discovered they enjoyed genital stimulation as a natural extension of non-genital pleasuring. Although shy at the beginning, they had a breakthrough and both enjoyed being orgasmic. In
fact, rather than doing a "quickie intercourse," Ruth preferred manually stimulating Kyle to orgasm. Kyle found oral stimulation of Ruth

was great for her arousal and lubrication. With this base of genital pleasuring, they were able to develop comfort and enjoyment with intercourse. Most couples do not progress as rapidly, but comfort with genital pleasuring and eroticism is a crucial ingredient in a sexual relationship.

Preparing for Genital Pleasuring

These exercises are suggestions and guidelines designed to help in the exploring and discovering process, not a cookbook which you must follow in minute detail. These are not rigid tests you must pass to prove your sexuality. The focus is becoming aware of genital feelings and accepting a broad-based, flexible approach to sexuality. This learning is facilitated through an open, honest exchange, which allows full acceptance of yourselves as sexual people and a sexual couple.

Each exercise is intended to take thirty to ninety minutes; however, this is flexible. You may want to separate parts of an exercise and do these independently. Some couples choose to devote more time to a specific exercise, to not switch roles during the exercise, to repeat part of an exercise such as genital touching with clothes on, or to value integrating non-genital and genital touch. Plan a relaxed time in which you will not be disturbed or feel hurried. Genital pleasuring is an integral step in accepting yourselves as a healthy sensual and sexual couple.

First Set of Exercises: Breast Stimulation

Before beginning, sit and talk for ten minutes about the highlights of your non-genital touching experiences, then discuss what you need in order to feel receptive and comfortable with genital touch. Remind your partner what you valued in the non-genital touching and how important it is to continue this pleasure-oriented sharing process.

Hold hands as you go to take a shower or bath. Soap and caress as before, with one addition: wash your partner's entire body. When you reach the genital areas, name each part aloud—penis, mons, scrotum, vagina. You might use your favorite slang words, such as "prick," "jinnie," "junior," or "clit." Feeling comfortable with sexual language, whether it be slang, proper, or your private sexual vocabulary, facilitates communication. If arousal occurs during the bath or shower, view it as a healthy, natural process; do not feel pressure to do something—simply accept it.

Dry each other, including the genital area, in the natural progression of drying from top to bottom. Do not save the genitals for last. Include them as a natural part of your partner's body.

Be sure the bedroom milieu is conducive to feeling sensuous and receptive. Are you comfortable with the lighting? Some people like it bright; others prefer a darker room. Do not make it so dark that you cannot see the details of your partner's nude body. If music puts you in a sensuous mood, then by all means play your favorite music on the radio, stereo, or DVD player.

The male initiates. Begin with a favorite position from the non-genital exercises which gives you access to your partner's body and breasts. With your right hand, gently caress her breasts as an extension of caressing her chest and sides. She can close her eyes to increase awareness of the rhythm and type of breast touch she finds particularly sensuous. She should not pressure herself into feeling sexually aroused nor should you try to arouse her. The role of the receiver is to be passive and allow herself to be receptive to and accepting of pleasure. The idea of being selfish and accepting sensual and sexual stimulation is difficult for some women—especially those who always worry about pleasing the partner and ignoring their needs and desires. It is important to be selfish in the sense of accepting pleasure. This facilitates developing a vital couple relationship. When you are open to receiving pleasure, you give more to your partner—this is the reciprocal function of the "give to get" guideline.

Both giver and receiver can think of her breasts as parts of her body to discover and explore. The man can view her breasts anew and feel comfortable in exploring a variety of touches and strokes. She can be aware and comfortable with her sensations and feelings.

Gradually focus on breast stimulation. With the palm of the hand, start at the waist and move up to the neck with one long motion. Be careful not to press hard; breasts can be sensitive and you might inadvertently cause discomfort. She is free to tell you if it hurts or if there is discomfort, and to request a different area or type of touch. Sometimes the difference between pleasurable and irritating touch is less than an inch or merely a minimal difference in pressure. Trace the nipple with your fingertips and see if it becomes erect. Notice the different sensations of an erect, as opposed to non-erect, nipple. As you caress her breasts, be aware of and respond to warm, sensuous feelings.

Place your hand on your partner's opposite side so that you nearly surround her with your arm and, in a slow, continuous movement, draw your hand over the soft skin underneath the armpit, across both breasts and slowly back again. As you pass over a breast, if the nipple is soft, gently caress it until it is erect. If erect, stop stimulation and see if it becomes soft.

Lift yourself on your elbow for support, kiss and caress her breasts and chest. Feel the texture changes with your tongue. Allow manual and oral stimulation to be gentle and non-demanding. Harder, focused, erotic stimulation is inviting if she is aroused, yet is counterproductive (or irritating) if she is not.

Throughout this exercise, the emphasis is on nonverbal communication since talking can get in the way of bodily feelings. As giver, be sensitive to any signs of tension or anxiety. If you feel her become tense, back off, but do not remove yourself from body contact; that is, keep the connection, but alter the touching. If kissing breasts makes her tense and you feel it or she reports it, move your kisses to her face, chest, or stomach until she is comfortable. Do not move away or cease contact. Neither of you has made a mistake. It takes time and experience to gain comfort and learn what is pleasurable. Intermix non-genital touch with breast stimulation. Stay with the feelings, enjoy the sense of exploration and discovery. Your openness helps your partner to be comfortable and feel receptive to the pleasuring.

After the male has given her a variety of experiences—including touching the areola with just the palm of his hands, gently bringing the breasts as close together as they will go, and exploring the difference in separate versus simultaneous breast stimulation—you can change roles.

Although the male has experienced breast stimulation during non-genital touching, focusing on the male breast in a sensual and sexual way is a new experience. Explore the difference in feeling between an erect and non-erect nipple and note how, or if, he enjoys having his nipples touched and kissed. Some men find this pleasurable, others do not. There are no right or wrong responses. The recipient is engaged in a process of discovering how his body reacts to stimulation. Express warmth by touching and kissing attractive parts of his body. End the pleasuring on a caring note.

Afterwards, sit and discuss each partner's feelings about breast touching—manual and oral. Some couples find breast stimulation is not their "thing." That also is acceptable. How would you like breast stimulation to fit into your sexual sharing? How can you increase pleasure and arousal?

Second Set of Exercises: Genital Exploration

Begin with a bath or shower. This time, while soaping your partner's genitals, describe verbally and in detail such things as skin appearance, size, and attractiveness. What do you find particularly fascinating about your partner's genitals? Use words for genitals—proper, slang, or your private sex language—whichever is most comfortable.

The woman begins as giver while he keeps his eyes closed. During the exercise, we suggest a minimum of verbal interaction. Focus on sensations and feelings. He lies on his back, his eyes closed, his body relaxed and passive. She assumes a comfortable position, perhaps kneeling near his stomach or sitting or lying beside him.

Visually explore his body. Allow your eyes to range over his entire body, not just the genitals. Spend time massaging and caressing your favorite non-genital body parts. As you do this, observe his genitals. Be aware of your feelings about an erect as opposed to flaccid penis. A commonly believed myth is that when the male has an erection, the woman must *do* something, either have intercourse or bring him to orgasm. An erection might indicate general excitement (often men feel this during a sports event or while wrestling with their children),

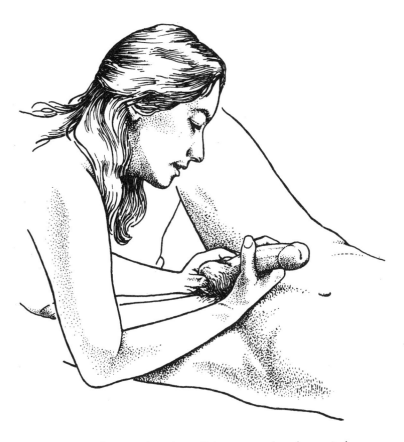

Nondemanding exploration of the external male genitals.

anticipatory sensual feelings, or sexual arousal. Interestingly, the male believes the myth that an erection *must* mean sexual arousal, and he attempts intercourse even when he does not feel like sex. This time do not do anything with the erection except enjoy it without feeling any demand.

While massaging around the stomach, lower your hand and touch his penis and scrotum. As you explore his genitals, be aware of each part you touch—penis, glans, shaft, frenulum, scrotum, testes. Touch and verbalize the parts until you feel comfortable. Touch the way you want—do a variety of playing, rubbing, and caressing. If either of you feels anxious, do not remove your hand, simply massage a body part which you feel comfortable with. Take a few long, deep breaths and allow yourself to relax. If you still feel anxious, hold your partner until the anxiety dissipates. Stay close; you are not in a sexual race. The giver can proceed at her pace and comfort level.

As you explore the testes, notice which is larger and what the shapes remind you of. Remember, these are sensitive body parts. Move slowly and gently. Notice how the testes move inside the scrotum.

If your partner is circumcised, trace the glans of the penis with your fingertips. If he is uncircumcised, gently move the foreskin back and explore the glans. Enjoy non-demand massage and caresses around the inner thighs, perineum, and scrotum. If he becomes erect, keep your hand on the penis and stroke it. Notice the pulse as blood collects in the penis and enjoy the feeling of it becoming erect. Place your hands in a cuplike curve and hold the scrotum. Notice how his scrotum changes as arousal intensifies. After his penis has been erect for a while, either move to non-genital touching or discontinue stimulation until the erection subsides. Erection naturally waxes and wanes (as does female lubrication). Note the differences in the penis and scrotum in the non-erect state.

The male should be aware of his feelings as his erection subsides. Males traditionally become anxious or panicked with the waning of an erection. Men are used to proceeding to intercourse and orgasm on their first erection. His erection waning is nothing to be anxious or threatened about. An erection decreases and is regained if the male

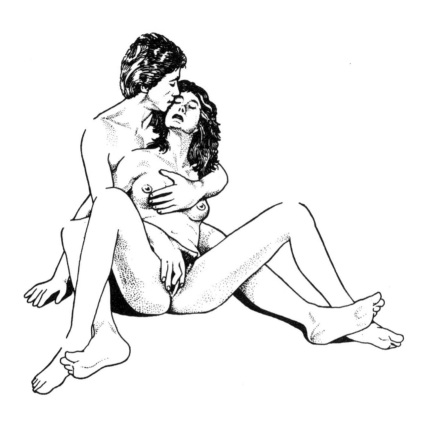

Nondemanding stimulation of the female genitals.

allows it to happen without overreacting with anxiety or making self-demands to will an erection. In a prolonged pleasuring/foreplay period, it is not unusual for an erection to wax and wane two to five times. Waxing and waning of erections is a natural physiological process. Males are unaware of this because their stereotyped pattern is to have an orgasm on their first erection.

Run your fingers through his pubic hair. Notice the texture, thickness, and length. With your fingertips trace a line down to his anus. Then, flattening your hand, caress the inside of one leg while you continue to hold and gently squeeze his penis. Try to coordinate the rhythm of his breathing with the stroking of his penis. Gently pull and squeeze at the same time. Place your other hand on his lower abdomen and caress with a circular movement.

The role of the giver is to provide a variety of stimulation so the receiver can discover what is pleasurable. At this point, only use manual touch. Oral genital stimulation can occur in subsequent experiences. When you feel comfortable with genital touch and have given your partner a pleasurable experience, switch roles.

The woman lies on her back and lets herself relax. The man can find a comfortable position, whether sitting, kneeling, or lying. It is important that he can see and touch her, especially her genitals. Begin by touching your favorite non-genital areas, and then let her guide your hands over her breasts by placing her hand over yours (the hand-over-hand technique). Let her teach you the type of breast touch which is most stimulating. She can tell you what pleases her by touch and gesture, or use verbal guidance if she prefers.

It is especially important to keep your communication process comfortable and clear. Learning is based on a positive influence process, not demands or intimidation. Repeat gestures or words so your partner understands and appreciates them. Sexual learning is a gradual process.

You might enjoy kissing, sucking, licking, tongue gliding or biting on the areola, nipple, or entire breast. She can guide by moving your head, touching your forehead, or a mutually understood gesture. Be careful as you kiss or suck because breasts can be sensitive—hard sucking is enjoyable only when she is aroused. Sensitivity and awareness enhance the experience for both.

Massage around the stomach, then explore her genitals. Gently run your fingers through her pubic hair and caress the mons. Be aware of the texture of her pubic hair and its appearance. Place the heels of both hands below her vulva in the soft inner part of her legs. With both hands cupped over her pubic hair, move them rhythmically in small circles.

Spread the labia majora with your fingers. Be comfortable with the sight and feel of her genitals. Identify the clitoris and clitoral shaft, and look carefully at the labia minora. Notice how the labia surround the vaginal introitus. Spread the vaginal opening with two fingers and notice the color and texture of the interior. Gently insert one finger into the vagina and notice the sensations of containment. Feel the warmth and dampness. Touch the mons, perineum, and around the urethra. As you explore, verbalize the names (using proper, slang, or your personal language).

Move slowly and gently. Allow tender touching and exploration to be sexually inviting. The clitoris can be especially sensitive, so rather than stimulating directly, run your fingers around the clitoral shaft. When she becomes aroused, her clitoris becomes enlarged and withdraws under the clitoral hood. This is her body's way of protecting itself from discomfort. Hard, direct clitoral stimulation causes pain for most women. Massage around the labia and clitoral shaft, thereby indirectly stimulating the clitoris.

Allow touching and exploring to be sensuous, tender, and caring. If she becomes aroused, lubricated, and responsive, remember to *respond* with her rather than feel the need to *do* something. Genital response and arousal is natural and normal, accept and enjoy it. Intermix non-genital touching—do not focus solely on genitals. When you are feeling comfortable with genital touch and have provided your partner with a variety of experiences, end the exercise in a warm, close manner.

Hold your partner, sharing feelings of tenderness and caring. Get dressed and go downstairs to talk or if you prefer, lie in bed. Share feelings; talk openly and frankly about genital exploration and touch.

Third Set of Exercises: Guiding

During this exercise, keep your eyes open and use eye contact to facilitate communication. Use your favorite lotion to enhance feelings of sensuality, remembering to warm it or pour it on your hand so it is warm before you rub it on your partner's skin. Use the hand-over-hand technique to guide and teach your partner the places and types of touch which give pleasure and increase responsiveness.

Couples often do not communicate how they like having their clothes taken off. Usually the man undresses himself and hastily undresses his partner. Begin with both partners dressed, and let the woman undress the man. She can start by looking at her partner fully clothed, then mentally undress him. Keep good eye contact with verbal interaction at a minimum so you can focus on the experience.

Begin undressing by playing in a teasing manner with the middle buttons on his shirt. Unbutton the shirt slowly; while doing so, put your hand on his crotch and notice his reaction. After you have taken the shirt off, you could unbuckle his belt and pants, turn him around, and lower his pants. Slowly take off shoes and socks and let him step out of his pants. Turn him around so he is facing you, look at him, and give him a big hug. Then take off his underpants. How do you feel about undressing him in a seductive, sensuous way? How did he feel? How does it feel to hug and kiss—her clothed, him nude?

The male can then undress the woman. First, do it visually. Then, kiss and hold her. Start in the middle of her back and run your finger up and down the zipper or buttons. Unzip or unbutton a little at a time, then stop and run your fingers up and down her back. Take one shoulder of her blouse off, stroking her arm. As you touch her back, check where the hooks on the bra are. Undo one strap at a time—do not take the bra off; just let it hang. Turn her around and take her shoes off. Next take off her skirt, or roll her slacks down slowly. Face each other— notice how she looks with her panties and loosely hanging bra. As you take off her bra and panties, say the warm sexy things you are feeling. When she is nude, take her in your arms and start the pleasuring.

In subsequent undressing experiences, vary these techniques according to your personal style—sometimes seductive, sometimes playful. Undressing can be sensuous, seductive, and fun rather than routine.

Decide who will begin. Whoever has more discomfort in *giving* should first be the giver. Attend to your partner's feelings and guidance. Remember the "give to get" guideline for mutual sexual satisfaction.

Try a different pleasuring position. The giver sits on the bed, with back support from the wall, bedboard, or soft pillows. The person's legs are spread far enough apart so the partner can sit between them.

The recipient might need back support, too. Arrange pillows to permit the receiver to be in a semi-reclining position. There is no set way to place the pillows; fix them so both people are comfortable. The recipient's legs will be over the giver's. Be sure the giver has full access to the receiver's entire body.

As giver, begin by caressing genitals, using your favorite lotion (be sure it is hypoallergenic). Go over the genitals as if your goal were to cover them completely with lotion. Do this slowly, tenderly, and rhythmically. Follow your partner's guidance. The receiver is free to guide his or her hands to parts of the genitals that feel particularly erotic and arousing.

Those who masturbate or have done self-exploration exercises are in a particularly good position to understand and share their natural bodily responses. Help your partner by making open, clear requests. Be there emotionally and sexually, share your pleasure.

When you are feeling aroused, switch to non-genital touching. Typically, touching goes quickly from non-genital to focused genital stimulation. How does it feel to reverse that process? Allow non-genital touch to be slow, tender, and rhythmic. Be responsive to your partner's guidance and feelings. Try to make non-genital touching as involving as genital touch. Guide your partner back to genital stimulation or your favorite combination of non-genital and genital. If you want, proceed to orgasm, but do not feel pressure to do so.

Switch roles and repeat the sequence. Afterward, lie in bed and share feelings. Discuss how you feel about giving as opposed to receiving. Do you like taking turns or doing mutual pleasuring? How do you feel about combining non-genital and genital touching? Be frank, direct, clear, and supportive. The most important thing to share is how you feel about yourselves as a sexual couple. Sexuality builds and reinforces intimate, loving feelings.

If you have difficulty talking about the experience or cannot express feelings of pleasure or dislike about specific activities, consider the following verbal exercise. This is more comfortably done clothed over the kitchen table, in the living room, or on a walk. If there has been a negative experience or you are giving difficult feedback, get up, get dressed, and talk outside the bedroom. Lying nude in bed is too vulnerable a position to deal with difficult feelings and issues. It is potentially explosive to share negative feelings in bed after a difficult sexual experience. The usual outcome is much heat, little light, and bruised feelings.

Choose an exercise you *can* comfortably talk about. There are no laws or rules dictating what exercises must be done in which order. Go back to a comfortable exercise and process it. Then discuss blocks and inhibitions, which interfere with sexual communication. Be aware that a difficult experience or miscommunication is not a personal rejection or due to malevolent intent. You are an intimate team trying to develop a respectful, trusting relationship and a comfortable, functional couple sexual style. If you have a good feeling you want to express but cannot, ask your partner about her or his feelings. Find a common ground of discussion where you can help each other express feelings and preferences. Do not make the mistake of bogging down on questions such as: "Am I really attractive?" "Can we be sexual?" "Do I deserve love?" These lead to a self-defeating, destructive cycle. Focus on specific issues and feelings which build sexual comfort and confidence.

Fourth Set of Exercises: Erotic Massage

The focus is on integrating genital and non-genital touch: oral, manual, and rubbing stimulation; using eye contact, hand guiding, and verbal feedback. During the first half of this exercise, engage in mutual touching with as much spontaneity and sharing as possible. Allow the exercise to be unstructured, with mutual giving and receiving.

The second part focuses on erotic massage. Return to giver-receiver roles and let the man be the giver first. The erotic massage integrates genital and non-genital touching. It is both sensual and sexual, involving caresses which are *slow, tender, caring, rhythmic,* and *flowing.*

The recipient lies on her stomach; her eyes can be open or closed, whichever feels more comfortable. Begin by massaging the back of her neck with both hands. Be sure her neck muscles are relaxed. Gently move your hands to about three inches above the tailbone and massage her upper and lower back in smooth, rhythmic motions.

Move your hands to the backs of the thighs and caress her buttocks. Bring your hands together at the small of the back; using the same motion, move to the thighs. Repeat this movement and be receptive to feelings of sensuality and eroticism.

Help your partner turn over. Gently place both hands on her thighs. With a smooth, sweeping movement, move your hands up her thighs and over the vulva; then bring them together at her stomach. Spread your hands in an outward movement toward both breasts. Bring her breasts together. Then with the same movement work the thighs. Be sure to touch the genitals fully. Integrate the pleasuring process. You might want to intermix manual and oral genital stimulation. Give your partner several different sexual caresses. Be aware of feelings of pleasure at your partner's enjoyment and responsiveness. Continue caressing until your partner requests you to stop. You can proceed to orgasm if you wish.

Change roles and let the woman repeat the same series of exercises. She can use her personal style of integrating pleasuring with an erotic massage.

There is an additional experience which can be particularly pleasurable. Typically, a woman will not use her breasts actively; instead, she is passive while the male stimulates them. Active breast stimulation can be enjoyable to the woman as well as her partner. After hand massage of the man's thighs, genitals, stomach, and chest, she can put lotion on her breasts and repeat the same movements using her breasts. Notice the feelings in your breasts; some women find breast responsiveness heightened during this experience. When you have done this long enough to determine whether it feels comfortable and arousing, have your partner lie comfortably on his side, put your hand on his chest, with your front to his back, and follow the rhythm of his breathing. This can be a warm, close, intimate feeling. Allow your-selves to breathe together and drift off to sleep.

Closing Thoughts

You can feel comfortable giving and receiving sensual and sexual stim-ulation in a non–goal-oriented atmosphere. You can develop a healthy attitude about yourself as a sexual person and yourselves as a sensual and sexual couple. Accept your sexuality and special style of giving and receiving pleasure. Non-genital and genital pleasuring is a solid foun-dation for sexual communication and functioning for your intimate relationship.

5

Self-Exploration and Masturbation

You are a sexual person from the day you are born to the day you die. Acceptance and enjoyment of sexuality varies depending on the individual, life experiences, values, and relationship. For some, sexual feelings develop naturally and at a young age; for others, sexual feelings and the acceptance of sexuality are delayed. Because of cultural factors, experiences, and expectations, some people develop positive sexual self-esteem and have a satisfying sexual life; others do not.

The purpose of these exercises is to increase knowledge of and comfort with your body and its natural, healthy responses. One way to remove blocks to naturally occurring sensual and sexual response is through a systematic, anxiety-reducing self-exploration of your body and its capacity for pleasure. This can improve your image of your body and build sexual self-esteem.

Orgasm

A major difference between men and women is how they learn about orgasm. Boys explore and touch their genitals earlier and more frequently. Typically, between ages ten and sixteen boys have their first orgasm, either through a nocturnal emission (wet dream) or self-stimulation (masturbation). They have a range of psychological reactions—

some boys are very pleased and see it as a passage into manhood; others are guilty and anxious; others feel excitement mixed with confusion or shame. Learning your body can react to stimulation with arousal and orgasm should be positive for both men and women.

Women tend to experience their first orgasm later than men, some through self-stimulation and others by partner stimulation. Less than 5 percent have their first orgasm during intercourse. Ten percent of adult women are non-orgasmic; in other words, they have not learned to experience the feeling of increasing excitement and responsivity followed by a moment of release (orgasm, climax) accompanied by a great deal of pleasure. All people have the potential to be orgasmic.

Physiologically and psychologically, orgasmic response is similar for men and women. Orgasm lasts from three to ten seconds and consists of rhythmic muscle contractions followed by the release of tension and vascular congestion in the pelvic area. A man typically experiences a single orgasm, which is accompanied by ejaculation. Women have the potential to experience multiple orgasms (about one in five women have multiple orgasms).

The media overdramatize the need and centrality of orgasm. Orgasmic experiences differ depending on the person, situation, and relationship. Orgasm has been described by some as a "pop," where tension has built and is replaced by a feeling of warmth and calm. Others have compared orgasms to waves—sometimes a gentle ripple, other times a roaring cascade in which the person might lose consciousness for a second or two.

Orgasm is a natural culmination of sexual responsivity and arousal. An orgasm cannot be willed or forced. The more you concentrate and strive for it, the less likely you are to experience orgasm. A healthy way to think about the process of arousal and orgasm is as a delightful heightening of pleasurable feelings beginning with sensual touching, moving into sexual arousal, and naturally culminating in intense sensations (orgasm) followed by afterplay. You can learn to be comfortable with your body and its sensual and sexual reactions, including being orgasmic.

Gail and Jack

Gail and Jack were experiencing sexual dysfunction. In reviewing their sexual histories, it was apparent attitudes and experiences with masturbation were a contributing factor.

Jack's problem was early ejaculation. He had begun masturbating at thirteen. Jack found masturbation and ejaculation very arousing, but was troubled by thoughts that he should not be doing this. He was afraid of being caught by his parents or discovered by his brother or sister. Jack vaguely remembered his father deriding an older neighborhood boy for "playing with himself" and vividly remembered the priest warning against the sin of "self-abuse." Jack developed a pattern of fast, intense, totally penis and orgasm-focused masturbation. He ejaculated as quickly as he could and cleaned up immediately so he would escape discovery. For Jack, masturbation and orgasm were intense, but not an integrated part of his life. As soon as he ejaculated, he wanted to forget about sex. This pattern extended to partner sex. Gail wanted a sensuous, slow, and tender lover, whereas Jack was genitally oriented, fast both in touching and intercourse, and abrupt in his movements. Gail misinterpreted this to mean he did not care about her. In fact, Jack valued their relationship; he was just repeating the pattern he overlearned during masturbation.

Slow, gentle body exploration was a central ingredient in treatment. If Jack could appreciate sensuality himself, it would be easier to share this with Gail. During masturbation exercises, Jack identified the point of ejaculatory inevitability and practiced extending ejaculatory control. As his comfort, skill and confidence improved, he transferred those learnings to sex with Gail.

Gail's experience with self-exploration and masturbation was quite different. She learned "good girls" were not to touch themselves "down there." Gail was not knowledgeable about her genital area and confused about the role of her clitoris. When she bathed and the stream of water ran over her vulva, there were positive sensations that caused ambivalent feelings. Gail felt similar ambivalence about her vagina. Her learning about menstruation was negative—she dreaded her monthly period. Boyfriends tried to touch and enter her vagina, and she became used to saying no. Gail's first intercourse was a disappointment. She was minimally lubricated, intromission was painful, and she felt cheated by the man not caring about her physical or psychological feelings. Sex with Jack added to her disappointment since his stimulation was rough, ejaculation was rapid, and sex ended with his orgasm. She felt Jack did not care about her sexual needs or feelings.

For Gail, developing comfort with her genitals and being responsible for learning her arousal and orgasm pattern constituted a new, challenging concept. Jack's support, especially taking care of children when she engaged in self-exploration and self-stimulation exercises, was of great value. Gail experienced initial discomfort, fearing she was "selfish." This was countered by realizing if she could become aware of her arousal and orgasm pattern, it would improve her sexual self-esteem and make their sexual relationship better. Gail discovered that touching her labia, stimulating her clitoral area, and using arousing fantasies allowed her to be orgasmic. As her comfort and confidence increased, she became an involved, active sexual partner.

Self-Exploration Guidelines

Each person is different, so consider the following as guidelines rather than rigid rules. You are a unique person; only you can know what is comfortable and arousing.

A first step is to increase comfort with and knowledge of your body. Set aside a time when you will not be interrupted. This is your time; do not answer the door and take the phone off the hook or put the answering machine on. If you have small children, use their afternoon nap time or put your spouse in charge of the house and children.

Remember three guidelines:

1. The focus is on exploration, learning, and comfort rather than the accomplishment of a specific goal. This is not a test with right or wrong answers.

2. Be flexible about time spent. Ideally, one set of exercises is done each time. The session can be from fifteen to sixty minutes. At first there might be embarrassment and hesitancy, which could cause you to stop prematurely, so try to have the first session at least ten minutes and allow them to become progressively longer.

3. Set up your surroundings to facilitate comfort and sensuality. Do you want the lights off or on? Do you want music? Do you like using oil, lotions, or powders? Make this a special time.

We have designed separate sets of exercises for men and women, although the concepts are very similar.

First Set of Exercises for Women:
Body Exploration

You need to be aware of and comfortable with your body. Make sure you have uninterrupted time and privacy. Draw a hot bath (or take a shower) and add your favorite bath oil. Stretch out in the tub and soap your body. Enjoy the sensations of your hands touching your calves, thighs, and arms. Spend time on your toes and feet, massaging them until they feel relaxed. Feel the softness behind your knees and on the inside of your upper arms. Cross your arms so opposite hands grasp your waist. Slide your hands across your body and down the sides to rest on your thighs. Sitting up, place your palms and knees together. Slide your hands through the thighs and caress your legs. Be aware of and responsive to your whole body. Lie back and relax. Dry yourself in a slow, comfortable manner, almost caressing yourself dry.

Go into the bedroom without clothes on and lie on your bed. You may want to darken the bedroom, turn up the heat, light a candle, have music on the radio or stereo. Do what is best for you. Use pillows to support yourself in the most comfortable position you can find.

Close your eyes and concentrate on relaxing. Be aware of any tension. The easiest way to discover and reduce tension is to tighten each muscle group (arms, legs, back, chest, face) in turn and then relax. To facilitate relaxation, repeat to yourself expressions like: "Relax,

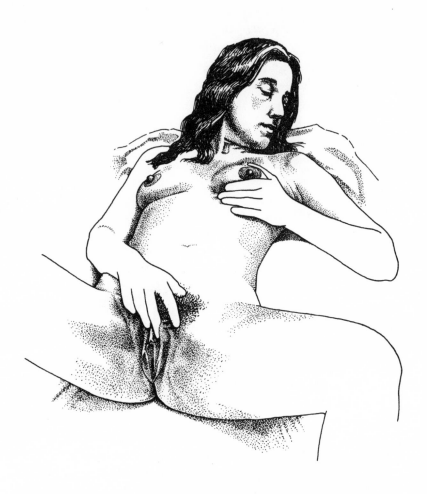

Self-exploration: an essential exercise in the discovery of your own
body's sensations.

and feel my body" or "Relax more and more, deeper and deeper." Use slow, deep, regular breathing to enhance relaxation. Each time you inhale, think the word "relax"; each time you exhale, think the word "calm."

When you are feeling relaxed and comfortable, gently clasp your thighs, curl up slowly and roll to one side. Notice the feelings of movement. Then touch your feet, legs, thighs, stomach, chest, lower back, neck, face, arms, and fingers. Try different types of touch—light stroking, patting, heavy massaging, rubbing, scratching. Be aware of sensations of touch on different parts of your body.

Take time for visual exploration. If possible, use a full-length mirror. An interesting technique is to take a piece of cardboard or paper, hold it first in front of one eye and then the other. Which parts of your body look different? Find at least one part which is different from its other side. Look at your whole body (front, side, and back views) and be aware of at least two areas you find particularly attractive (these do not have to be genital areas).

View your genitals with a small hand mirror as you lie on the bed or lie facing a full-length mirror with pillows propped under your buttocks. Identify parts of your vulva. Be comfortable with the sight and feel of your genitals. Do not be concerned about sexual arousal. Separate the labia majora with your fingers; look carefully at the labia minora and find the clitoris under its hood. Notice how the labia minora surrounds the vaginal opening. Spread the vaginal introitus with two fingers and notice the color and texture of the interior. Insert a finger into your vagina and watch with the mirror. Be aware of the warmth, softness, and dampness. How does it feel? Touch the mons area, the perineum (the area between the vagina and the anus), and around the urethra.

Close your eyes. Touch all the areas again, imagining how they look in the mirror. Develop comfortable, positive feelings about your body and genitals.

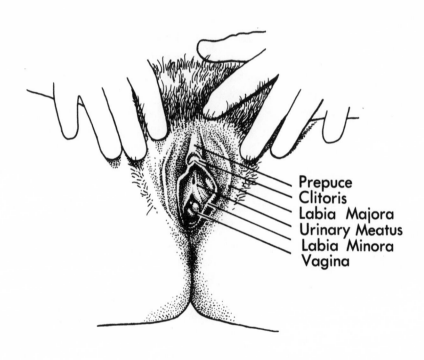

Prepuce
Clitoris
Labia Majora
Urinary Meatus
Labia Minora
Vagina

The genital anatomy of the female.

Key to Diagram:

MONS. A raised area created by a layer of fat over the pubic bone. The mons becomes covered with hair at puberty.

LABIA MAJORA. The literal translation is "greater lips."

LABIA MINORA. These folds of sensitive tissue become engorged as blood flows into them when you are sexually aroused.

PREPUCE. This hoodlike fold of tissue is formed by the joining of the labia minora. The prepuce covers the clitoris.

CLITORIS. This is the most sensitive and responsive part of your genitalia. It becomes enlarged and erect when stimulated. The clitoris is the organ with the most nerve endings and has no other function than sexual pleasure.

URINARY MEATUS. This is the outlet for urine from the bladder.

VAGINA. This organ is about four or five inches long. Its walls normally touch each other, but during intercourse they stretch considerably, and of course greatly stretch during childbirth. The vagina receives lubrication from mucus secretions when you are aroused. A thin elastic membrane, the *hymen*, partially covers the opening of the vagina. The hymen can be broken or stretched in a number of ways. The outer third of the vagina is the most sensitive, although sensitivity varies from woman to woman. The *pubococcygeal (PC) muscle* is about two finger joints inside the vagina. The anterior wall of the vagina, especially when firmly stimulated while aroused, is particularly erotic for many women (this has been labeled the "G" spot).

Second Set of Exercises: Sexual Exploration

Begin by taking a long, relaxing bath. Get used to the feeling of caressing your body and notice things you may not have been aware of. Exactly where is that mole? How does it feel to touch it? How does it feel to pat your shoulders gently? How does your body feel after you stop stroking?

The bath serves two functions: to help you relax and to clean your body. Using a mild hypoallergenic soap, gently cleanse your genitals. Separate the labia with your fingers and clean it to remove secretions.

Two sensitive subjects should be mentioned. First, whether you keep or cut genital hair is your preference. Some women shave; most do not. Make your decision to suit your comfort and taste (be aware of your partner's feelings), not some ideal promoted by the depilatory and razor industries. Second, everybody has odors. We suggest you cleanse odor-causing substances, but in doing so we are not advocating you give up your humanity to the soap and perfume manufacturers. Genital cleanliness is a sign of consideration for your partner, but some women find such sanitization unnatural and unappealing.

Feel your clitoris and gently wash your clitoral area. Take extra time to dry your body. Some women prefer a soft towel to caress themselves, others choose a stiff terrycloth for a stimulating massage while drying.

Do the modes of touching that you enjoy; allow yourself to be inventive. Feel comfortable with genital touch. Start by touching your breasts. When you slowly move one hand up the opposite side of your body, then over your chest, the areola will rise. Notice the difference in feeling when the areola is hard and when soft. Touch your breasts, be aware which is more responsive. What is the most enjoyable form of breast stimulation—stimulating concurrently? touching the areola with just the palm of your hand? rubbing downward on the breast and then pulling up? Women vary in their responsivity. Some very much enjoy having their breasts caressed; others do not. What are your responses and feelings?

Curl up on your side. Slide your hands up the inside of your legs until they reach the genital area. Run your fingers through your pubic hair. Feel the soft skin covering the area between your vagina and anus: this is the perineum. Be aware of the labia majora. Separate the lips, and with your fingertips touch and outline the labia minora. Find the clitoris, and placing a finger above it, slide back the clitoral hood. This is a small movement; at first you may have a hard time identifying your clitoris. Do you enjoy direct or indirect clitoral stimulation?

What type of touch and pressure feels best? Trace the outer edge of the vaginal opening with your fingertip. Notice that it becomes damp, moist, and warm. This normal body secretion is clean and germ-free. It is natural, positive, and necessary. Vaginal secretions reflect healthy responsiveness. You might want to take a drop on your fingertip, put it on your tongue and taste it.

Become aware of the pubococcygeal (PC) muscle. The PC muscle affects intravaginal sensations and can be strengthened by doing exercises. The easiest way to locate this muscle is to stop your flow while urinating. The muscle you use is the PC muscle.

Practice exercising the PC muscle. Tighten the PC muscle, hold for three seconds, and release. Repeat this exercise ten times in succession—it will only take a minute. Some women use PC exercises to increase vaginal awareness and sensitivity. Some women tense and contract the PC muscle during intercourse to heighten sensations and feelings.

If at any time you feel anxious or uncomfortable, do not stop completely or remove your hands. Move back a step until you again feel comfortable, focus on relaxation and pleasure. There is no rush; proceed at your own pace. Gradually you will become comfortable and enjoy your natural body responses.

Third Set of Exercises:
Enhancing Sexual Pleasure and Arousal

As knowledge and comfort increase, you may skip some steps. Continue exploring and learning, with a focus on enhancing feelings of pleasure and responsiveness. You have a right to feel erotic and to bask in feelings of pleasure and arousal.

Enjoy the freedom of owning every feeling you have. You might try using imagery, fantasy, or pictorial, written, Internet or video material to facilitate arousal. What kinds of fantasies turn you on? Fantasies can enhance desire and arousal. You might visualize yourself running free and naked on a beach. Imagine your partner saying you are the best lover in history. Fantasize having sex for three hours, being stimulated by two lovers simultaneously, having sex with forbidden partners in exotic places—anything that turns you on. Give free reign to your fantasies and utilize them to enhance desire and arousal.

Most women find clitoral stimulation particularly arousing. Start with non-genital touching, and as you begin to feel receptive and responsive, move your hand to the clitoris and let your finger move across it slowly, back and forth. This can produce intensely erotic feelings. As you become aroused, your clitoris becomes engorged and withdraws under the clitoral hood. This is your body's way of protecting you from discomfort. Massage around the clitoral shaft, thereby indirectly stimulating the clitoris. Enjoy feelings of sensuality, eroticism, and arousal. If at any time you become anxious or uneasy, relax; move back a step, focus on the sense of comfort, and then return to stimulation. While massaging the vagina, take the secretions and spread them throughout the vulva. Spread the vaginal opening with two fingers and notice the texture of the interior. Feel the warmth and dampness. Insert a finger into your vagina and be aware of your feelings. Move your finger inside the vagina and study the sensations. Be aware of special places and feelings. When aroused, some women find anterior wall ("G" spot) stimulation highly arousing, others prefer clitoral stimulation. What is your responsivity/arousal pattern?

You can focus attention on the clitoral area or massage the clitoral shaft while caressing a breast with your other hand. Or you can combine clitoral and vaginal stimulation while focusing on sexual fantasies. Do what gives you the most erotic feelings. As arousal builds, go with it, and if it naturally culminates in orgasm, fine. If arousal does not result in orgasm, that is fine, too, since you are learning to increase awareness and responsivity.

Fourth Set of Exercises:
Building and Reinforcing Arousal

Experience your body as an integrated sensual and sexual whole. There is no longer an artificial barrier between touching your genitals and the rest of your body. You can facilitate the process by repeating sentences like these as you relax and touch: "Relax and enjoy my body"; "Find what feels good"; "Let go and feel it all."

Give yourself permission to enjoy sensual and sexual feelings. Some days certain scenarios and techniques feel particularly good; other days they do not. Discover the areas and touches that are a turn-on; be conscious of the pattern and rhythm to which you are most responsive. Experiment with different types of stroking (circular, upward, patting, quick touch, slowly building, rhythmic, teasing). Try variations in pressure to discover what is most stimulating. Stroke your clitoris with one hand while touching your breast or inner thigh with the other. Try massaging the clitoral shaft with one hand and intravaginal stimulation with the other.

You might want to entertain explicit sexual fantasies or read erotic material; do whatever would enhance sexual responsiveness. You might imagine making love with the sexiest man you ever saw. Imagine being sexual in a variety of exotic situations. Think about a favorite passage from an erotic poem or watch a sexual video. Fantasizing is not only normal, it is a healthy bridge to sexual desire and arousal.

You might experiment with the use of a vibrator to enhance arousal. Try an electric two-speed handheld vibrator with rubber attachments. Play with the vibrator on non-genital areas to become accustomed to the sensations. Then spread your knees, begin at the thighs, and move the vibrator slowly until it is resting against your labia. Spread the labia with your fingers and gently place the vibrator close to your clitoris. Experiment with placement until you find a sensitive part of your clitoral area and allow the vibrator to provide stimulation. As arousal builds, move your pelvis in rhythm with erotic sensations. When you experience the physical and emotional release of orgasm, accept it as the natural culmination of your body's receptivity and responsivity.

When you experience orgasm, you have taken a major step in acceptance of yourself as a sexual person and can share these learnings with your partner.

Closing Thoughts: Women

The exercises are designed to help you experience your body in sensual and sexual ways and to increase awareness of natural, healthy responses. You may or may not be orgasmic. If you are experiencing orgasm, congratulations. You have taken a major step. If not, do not be discouraged. These exercises involve one step in learning sensual and sexual responsiveness. You have taken a crucial step; you have become aware and accepting of your body. In time, practice, discovery, and reinforcement of the feelings and stimulation that you find sexually arousing will carry you to orgasm. If you keep enjoying and exploring with your partner and by yourself, you will achieve sexual arousal, which will culminate *naturally* in orgasm.

First Set of Exercises for Men:
Body Exploration

Begin with a bath or shower. Soap your body in a leisurely fashion, gently massage the larger muscle groups: arms, shoulders, neck, back, thighs, and calves. Spend time on your toes and feet. Keep massaging until they are relaxed. Be aware of the muscle tension in each body part. Healthy muscle has natural tension which does not interfere with relaxed feelings. Anxiety and stress cause muscle tension and produce uncomfortable, tight feelings which you can identify and relax away.

Allow anxiety and tension to drain from your body and replace it with feelings of calm and comfort. Let go and allow your muscles to relax. Be aware of physical feelings of warmth, heaviness, and comfort and psychological feelings of calm, confidence, and control.

The coarse spray of a shower provides a good massage. Soak in the warmth. Turn your face into the spray, which can massage and relax the muscles of your face. Bow your head and let the water run over your head, face, and neck. Let your worries, concerns, or embarrassments drain away so you can respond to the sensations of your body. Learning to feel relaxed and comfortable at first takes focus, as it is not something males in our culture learn. This is your time—enjoy it!

When you are feeling comfortable and relaxed—not when you *think* you *should be* feeling that way—get out of the shower and enjoy the feeling of your wet, dripping body. Notice the cooling sensation of water evaporating from your skin. As you dry, use the towel to give yourself a comfortable rubdown.

Go to the bedroom in the nude and sprawl on your bed. Be sure the bedroom is warm. Make the room as comfortable as possible. Do what you prefer; put your favorite music on the stereo or radio and darken the room if you wish.

Settle back on the bed; close your eyes and relax. Be aware of any tension in your body. The easiest way to identify tension is to tense muscle groups (arms, legs, back, chest, face) and then relax and release the tension. Prolong the feelings by letting your muscles relax even more. To facilitate and enhance feelings of relaxation, breathe deeply and regularly for two minutes. Each time you inhale, think the word "relax"; each time you exhale, think the word "calm." You might repeat to yourself expressions like: "Relax and feel my body"; "Let go completely"; or "Relax more and more, deeper and deeper."

When you are feeling relaxed, double up in a ball and roll to one side. Notice the feelings as you move. Begin touching yourself slowly and gently, first touching non-genital areas. Touch your feet, legs, thighs, stomach, chest, lower back, neck, face, arms, and fingers. Experiment with and be aware of different sensations from light stroking, rubbing, gentle patting, light touching, and heavy massage. Change positions and enjoy sensuous feelings.

Take time for visual exploration. Look at yourself in the mirror (a full-length mirror is preferable). Take a piece of cardboard or paper and place it in front of one eye (or simply close one eye). Examine half of your body, then switch; cover the other eye and examine the other half. Find at least one body part that does not look the same on both sides. Then look at your whole body (front, side, and back views) with both eyes and be aware of at least two non-genital areas you particularly like.

Thus far, we have emphasized non-genital touching and looking because males put undue emphasis on their genital anatomy. For

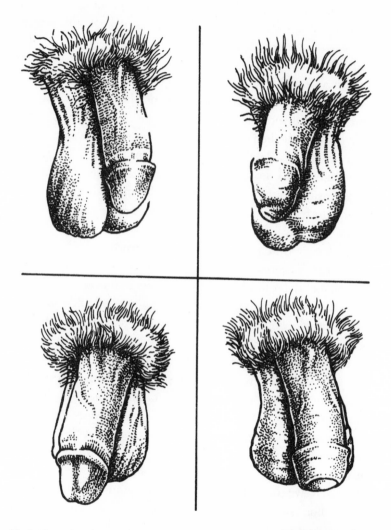

Variations in size and shape of external male genitals: Figures on the left show penises of circumcised males; those on the right, of uncircumcised males.

example, three-quarters of males worry their penis is smaller than average. Myths about penis size and its relationship to sexual prowess abound, and are blatantly false.

Be comfortable with the sight and feel of your genitals rather than worrying about sexual arousal. Touch the glans of the penis, frenulum, coronal ridge, and underside of the penile shaft. Examine your scrotum and discover which testis is larger. Notice how one testis is lower than the other, and be aware of the sensitivity of the scrotal sac. Observe the placement and feeling of your genitals while standing, sitting, or lying down. Close your eyes and touch the areas again, imagining how they look. Be aware of what parts of your body feel most comfortable and relaxed. End the exercise when you feel comfortable with your body and genitals.

Second Set of Exercises: Sexual Exploration

Enhance awareness of sensual and sexual feelings. Start with a shower or bath; this has the twofold purpose of cleansing your body and helping you relax. While showering or bathing, be aware of body hair. What places are hairy and which are hairless? How does your beard feel to the touch? Notice particularly the hair in your armpit and pubic area, and be sure to wash them. Body secretions and smells can be sensuous and sexually arousing; however, body odor caused by not washing is not attractive for you or your partner. Smell the natural scent of your body. If you use deodorant, talc, cologne, or other products, choose one that has an inviting scent.

Go nude into your bedroom and make yourself comfortable. Begin sensuous touching. Explore touching your breasts. Some men find breast stimulation enjoyable and arousing, others have no particular sensations. Watch your nipples and notice differences when they are soft and hard; note how they become erect and hard when you massage them. What are your feelings?

Lying on the bed, place your hands on your knees and slide them upward along the inside of your thighs; note the changes in sensitivity as you approach your genital area. Notice, too, how the hair on your legs thins out until the front of your upper thighs is nearly hairless. Enjoy the feeling of running your fingers through your pubic hair. Touch and massage the soft skin that covers the area between your genitals and anus—this is the perineum which can be quite sensual.

If at any time you feel anxious or self-conscious, do not stop. Move your hand to a body area where you feel comfortable. Take your time and move at your own pace. This is meant to be an exploring and learning experience; do not pressure yourself to feel arousal. Increase awareness of and comfort with your natural body reactions so that you can share them with your partner.

Now move your hand to your genitals. Discover what type of penile touch is most enjoyable and arousing. Be aware of feelings in touching your penis when it is flaccid as opposed to erect. Experiment with different types of genital touching; touch your penis using two fingers around the glans, put your hand around the shaft and stroke, let one hand touch your testicles and the other massage the frenulum, or employ any type of stimulation you enjoy. Be aware how much pressure on the shaft is most pleasurable. Play with different rhythms of penile stroking. Carry this to ejaculation if you desire, but do not feel pressure to do so. What kind of genital touching do you find most arousing? Continue self-stimulation until you feel comfortable with your pattern of genital responsivity.

Third Set of Exercises:
Sexual Pleasure, Arousal, and Orgasm

As you become comfortable with your body's sensual and sexual responses, focus on specific feelings of pleasure, eroticism and arousal. In order to guide your partner and teach her your arousal pattern, you must learn it for yourself. Make the milieu as comfortable as possible in terms of lighting, music, and atmosphere. To increase feelings of desire and arousal, do not hesitate to use written, Internet or visual materials. Many men find arousal increases by looking at pictures from *Playboy* or *Penthouse,* sex videos, reading erotic novels, sex magazines, love poems, pornography, or letters from their partner. Experiment and discover what is most arousing for you. Remember, there are no right or wrong, normal or abnormal methods of stimulation. Whatever feels sexually arousing is healthy as long as it is not compulsive and is transferable to partner sex.

Fantasizing can greatly increase feelings of desire and arousal. Some men fantasize having intercourse with a movie star, many fantasize about exotic positions and situations, and others about group sex or dominant-submissive scenarios. Feel free to employ fantasies that arouse you. Do not worry about their content: fantasy and behavior are different domains. There is no such thing as an abnormal fantasy as long it does not become obsessive or guilt-ridden. Guilt and obsessiveness result in a pattern by which fantasies become narrow, compulsive and self-defeating.

Begin touching with a focus on sensual feelings. A major trap males fall into is making masturbation a rapid, strictly genitally-oriented and orgasm-directed experience. This can result in a pattern of early ejaculation during couple sex. Slow down and enjoy the eroticism, arousal, orgasm process. Notice the feelings in your genitals and whole body as arousal increases. Focus on the type of stimulation that increases arousal and allows you to be orgasmic (i.e., orgasm triggers). This might be a slow, gradually increasing movement of your hand along the shaft of the penis, rubbing the area around the frenulum and glans, one hand massaging the scrotum while the fingers of your other hand manipulate the glans. Do what is most arousing for you.

When you ejaculate, be aware of the pleasurable feelings of sexual release. Enjoy your sexual arousal cycle. Be aware and accepting of your semen. You might want to look at the semen, touch it, and perhaps even taste it. It is a natural, positive aspect of you. Allow yourself to bask in the healthy, natural feelings of your body and sexual responsivity.

Fourth Set of Exercises: Integration

Focus on integrating sensual and sexual stimulation. Experiment with different techniques of self-stimulation to increase awareness of the variety of experiences available. Do not fall into the trap of making your touching completely genitally- or orgasm-oriented.

Enhance your mood by using music, reading material, relaxation, lighting, atmosphere. Begin with sensual whole-body touch before focusing on your genitals and penis. You might experiment with a lotion to increase sensations. Feel free to use erotic fantasies or materials.

Rather than utilizing touch as the only form of stimulation, try a different means of arousal. Turn over and rub your penis against the sheets of the bed, perhaps against a blanket or pillow between your legs. Feel the sensations on your thighs, buttocks, and chest. Feel your entire body as you stroke and enjoy feelings in your scrotum and penis. Focus on the most enjoyable type and amount of genital pressure. Consistent stimulation builds the urge to ejaculate. You might experiment with a stop-start manner of stimulation. Be aware of the point of ejaculatory inevitability, the period one or two seconds before orgasm begins. Allow yourself to experiment with and experience different types of penile stroking and massaging (circular, patting, heavy touch, light touch). Let yourself go and feel the maximum in sensuality and sexuality as you experience the healthy arousal and response of your body.

Closing Thoughts: Men

Self-exploration and masturbation exercises allow you to experience your body in sensual and sexual ways. You can be comfortable with your whole body and its natural, healthy responsiveness, rather than attention focused only on your penis and the three to ten seconds of orgasm. With increased awareness and comfort, it will be easier to share with your partner. A mixture of sensual non-genital touching and genital touching enhances pleasure and arousal during partner sex. Goal-oriented sexual experiences are less satisfying than sensual, pleasurable, erotic, mutually arousing experiences that naturally flow into and culminate in orgasm. You have taken an important step toward understanding and accepting your sexuality.

III

Enhancing Sexual Satisfaction

6

Non-Demand Pleasuring:
The Key to Sexual Intimacy

One of the most widely believed and harmful myths is that all touching must, and should, end in intercourse. Sexual expression is crippled by the idea that you cannot just be affectionate or enjoy playful touch, that any physical intimacy is an invitation to intercourse. Spontaneous affection and sensual touching turn into a demand for a goal-oriented sex performance.

Spontaneity and sharing increase when you are free to express feelings and affection without any expectation or demand other than the enjoyment of being together. You can enjoy touching in a non-demanding atmosphere, both inside and outside the bedroom.

Sexual pleasure is enhanced if you feel free to engage in affectionate touching and sensual pleasuring. This increases warm, caring feelings. It serves as a bridge to sexual desire, which might be crossed at that time or later. However, the bridge is blocked if touching is seen as a demand for intercourse. The key to a vital and satisfying sexual relationship lies in the value that both partners place on incorporating intimacy, non-demand pleasuring, and eroticism.

Sharing Thoughts and Feelings

Much stress and confusion exist because people do not share how they feel about being together—how much they enjoy being close and affectionate, when they want to be playful but not sexual. If your sexual relationship is based on the myth that satisfaction lies only in both partners' orgasm, or the even more harmful myth that simultaneous orgasm should be the goal, this perfectionist performance pressure subverts sexuality. It is fine to be orgasmic, or even orgasmic simultaneously, but to overemphasize the idea that intercourse and orgasm *must* happen is dangerous. This negates spontaneity and puts stringent demands on what should be an enjoyable, free-flowing experience.

The couple that develops a comfortable style of giving and receiving pleasure and sharing intimacy in a non-demand atmosphere will enhance sexual desire, functioning, and satisfaction. When intercourse and orgasm become the criteria for success, the sexual relationship loses. Mutual sharing and satisfaction are healthy criteria. You can share a fulfilling intimacy simply by being together and engaging in affectionate touch, sensual stimulation, and/or playful sexuality. With this non-demand attitude and pleasure orientation you both win; it is not a competition in which one partner wins and one loses.

Touching

Touching is integral to an intimate relationship. Touching allows both partners to express feelings of warmth and caring. Spontaneous touching in non-demand positions and situations, without an expectancy that sexual intercourse *must* follow, keeps a relationship free. With this open attitude come affection, sensuality, sexual desire, and intercourse. If you desire to proceed to intercourse, the decision is free-flowing, cued by involvement and arousal rather than by the feeling "We've gone this far—we have to go all the way."

A helpful and motivating metaphor for touching involves "five gears." First gear is clothes-on, affectionate touch (holding hands, kissing, hugging). Second gear is non-genital sensual touch, which may be done clothed, semi-clothed, or nude (body massage, cuddling on the couch, showering together, touching while going to sleep or on awakening). Third gear is playful touch, which intermixes genital and non-genital touching, clothed or unclothed, and may take place in bed, while dancing, in the shower, or on the couch. Fourth gear is erotic touch (manual, oral, or rubbing) leading to arousal and orgasm for one or both partners. Fifth gear integrates pleasurable with erotic touch and flows into intercourse.

Non-demand touching does not have to occur principally in bed or even in the bedroom. Keeping a relationship fresh and spontaneous involves a willingness to experiment with touching in a variety of times, places, and situations. It is inappropriate to engage in sexually arousing touching in a public place such as a street corner, but being sexual on a deserted beach, during a walk in a wooded area, or in a car parked by a lake adds spice to your relationship. More comfortable is the privacy of your house—using all the rooms, including the rug in front of the fireplace, the big chair in the living room, the dining-room table, or even the kitchen floor.

One variation to explore in such pleasuring is with clothing. Most sexual encounters involve nudity. This is fine, yet why limit it in that manner. The woman who appears wearing only a shirt can be quite enticing, as can the man wearing only his pants (or vice versa). We dress attractively when in public—what about dressing attractively, seductively, or playfully for your partner?

Another interesting and exciting variation involves positioning. There is no right or normal position for sexual activity. We suggest pleasuring positions to facilitate exploration. We also suggest experimentation with intercourse positions, initiation patterns and the way intercourse plays out.

Non-demand pleasuring keeps spontaneity, experimentation, and communication alive in your relationship. The couple that enjoys affectionate exchanges such as kissing, holding hands, and hugging has a solid intimate base. This is enhanced by sensual experiences such as showering together, head or foot massages, whole body massages with lotion, or dancing semi-clothed—all of which are both valuable in themselves and as bridges to sexual desire.

Jean and David

Jean and David have been married twenty-two years. They feel satisfied with their sexual relationship now more than ever. The last of their two children is about to leave for college, and they are looking forward to "being a couple again."

Although not a "feely-touchy" couple in public or at parties, they are warm and affectionate in private. Both are busy, but consciously set aside couple time without the distractions of children, household tasks, bills, or practical decisions. This time is spent taking walks, having a glass of wine or cup of tea while sitting on the porch, lying in bed talking and caressing, or going out for a cup of coffee and dessert. Their talk is about ordinary things, but each knows if there were something personal or difficult to be discussed, the spouse would be receptive. Typically, couple time involves affectionate and playful touching. Depending on moods and circumstances, about one-third of the time they proceed to intercourse. David and Jean have learned to communicate what they want and do not want sexually. The majority of their sexual activities is mutually involving and culminates in intercourse. When Jean is not aroused and does not feel like a "quickie" (why drip afterward is her rationale), she will stimulate David to orgasm. This does not feel like "mechanically doing" David, but "giving" to him and enjoying his arousal. When Jean is aroused and wants to be orgasmic but David is not feeling sexually desirous, he is open to giving her oral stimulation. Occasionally, they get signals crossed and have a "blah" or unpleasant experience. They accept that, laugh it off, and try again the next day when they are feeling more receptive and desirous. They hold to a forty-eight-hour rule that if they have a frustrating or failure experience, they will do something sensual or sexual within two days rather than let negative thoughts and feelings build.

First Set of Exercises:
Communicating Alternatives

Discuss feelings about non-demand touching. Be aware when and how you feel sexual pressure that diminishes spontaneity and mutuality. In these exercises, there is no demand—your desires and choices are what count. Develop and refine a "signal system" which tells your partner whether you desire to proceed to intercourse. This communication may be verbal, such as "I really want to make love," "I'm not in the mood to screw," "Let's get it on," "Let me just hold you," or "I've enjoyed this, let it be." The communication could be nonverbal, for example massaging your partner's genitals and switching to an intercourse position, moving to sensuous pleasuring, using eye contact to say yes or no, or moving your partner's hands to or from your genitals. Your partner has a signal that says "Okay," or "Not tonight—let's just play." Don't stop at "no"; suggest something you would like to engage in: a backrub, lying and talking, holding each other, a sensuous bath, giving manual or oral sex, taking a walk.

For this exercise, be nude in the bedroom. Lying on the bed, the woman positions herself behind her partner with their entire bodies touching, her chest to his back, her knees bent inside his. Her arms are around his body while he holds her hands. This is a nice position in which to lie together and feel connection and closeness. He is in a protected and passive position, allowing himself to feel cared for.

It is the woman's prerogative to indicate whether she wants to extend pleasuring into intercourse. She can use any signal system she wants, verbal or nonverbal; the criterion of effectiveness is whether he clearly receives and understands the communication. If her signal is positive, he can say whether he also desires intercourse. Couples make a mistake in assuming that the male always wants intercourse and must accede to her initiation. This sets unrealistic and demanding expectations and pressures. It is optimal when both partners feel comfortable initiating intercourse and both have the right to say no. If the man does not desire intercourse, he can suggest an alternative he would like. One possibility is to hold each other and talk. Another might be manually or orally stimulating her to orgasm. Another is engaging in whole-body pleasuring. If the woman signals she does not desire intercourse, she suggests an alternative sensual or erotic experience. One possibility is to sleep in this position, another to stimulate him manually or orally, a third to engage in mutual genital stimulation which could proceed to orgasm for one or both. If one or both become highly aroused, the usual pattern is to go to intercourse. This is especially true when you have just recently become a sexual couple; newness and frequency of sex are the focus. This is fine, but it is not a realistic model for sex in ongoing relationships. Nothing bad happens if arousal does not culminate in orgasm. Sexual expression is a choice, not a demand.

Discuss this experience in the morning, focusing on how comfortable and clear your communication system was. If there was a problem, what would you be willing to try next time to improve the communication process and sexual experience? Be aware there are a number of affectionate, sensual, playful and erotic alternatives (remember the five-gear metaphor). It is not a matter of intercourse or nothing.

Second Set of Exercises: Change of Setting

Are you as comfortable initiating intercourse as having a sensual experience? Does your partner accept your request or change it to something more enjoyable? If you decide not to continue to intercourse, are there feelings of pressure, grumbling or rejection? If there are difficulties or miscommunication, feel free to repeat the first exercise or use the same roles (female initiating, male responding) with this set of exercises. If things went well last time, let the male decide whether to continue to intercourse.

Choose a place other than the bedroom. It can be the living room, den, guest bedroom, bathroom, basement, or anywhere he chooses. This exercise is best done in the nude so you can be comfortable with nudity outside the bedroom. Be sure you will not be disturbed by children. Being affectionate in front of children and with children is positive. However, engaging in provocative or erotic activity in front of children is not healthy for adults or children. Sexuality involves privacy, comfort, and personal space. Children who grow up in families surrounded by overt sexuality find themselves as adults no less uncomfortable as those from families where there was no touching or communication about sexuality.

The man lies on his stomach, arms extended over his head. He can use cushions or pillows to rest his arms on. Lying on her side, the woman covers his arms and with one hand holds his. Her other hand is free to caress his back. One leg is placed over his for more contact. This position allows her to touch and caress his body; he can be passive or return the caresses. Since males have the tendency to become active and initiating, she may have to remind him this is a non-demand position where the pleasuring and caressing comes from her. This position—as other non-demand positions—can be reversed with the man covering, holding, and caressing her.

It is the man's prerogative to decide whether to continue to intercourse and orgasm. He can use a signal system, verbal or nonverbal, to communicate whether he wants to continue nondemand pleasuring or proceed to intercourse. The male needs to be attentive to his feelings and desires. If he signals for intercourse, it is not because he should or is expected to, but because he wants to. Likewise, the female responds with what she really wants rather than with what he wants or what she "should" do, not fearing disapproval or repercussions. Many women have come to view the male's erection as a demand for sex rather than a sign of pleasure and enjoyment. Couple sexual functioning improves when both partners are aware of feelings and desires, and communicate clearly and directly. If desires are different, it is easier to resolve by suggesting an alternative sensual or erotic activity rather than just saying no. If you communicate, you will usually discover a way of proceeding which is good for both.

Third Set of Exercises: Undressing

You are developing a growing awareness of the benefits of non-demand pleasuring. It enhances sexual intercourse when you decide to continue, and can be an affirmation of you as an intimate couple when you choose to remain sensual, to be playful, or to engage in erotic, non-intercourse sex. To make non-demand pleasuring more like your real-life sexual relationship, it is worthwhile to experiment with the amount of clothing as well as locations.

Begin by slowly or teasingly disrobing your partner to a state of undress (other than nudity) that you find to be the most appealing. Undress your partner in a manner that is seductive or playful. Some women find their man most enticing when he is wearing only underpants. Others like him fully clothed on top and nude on the bottom. Do what you like. Some males like their partners best in an

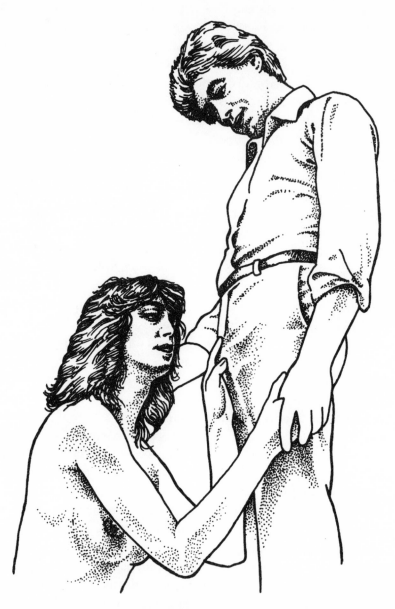

Non-demand touching of a clothed partner: an effective exercise in maintaining sexual intimacy.

unbuttoned blouse and panties or nude on the bottom and wearing the man's shirt and a headband. Your personal tastes are what is important.

The man can sit propped on pillows with his legs spread. Facing him she lies between his spread legs, with her knees near the side of his body. She can have pillows for the lower back so she is in a comfortable position to look and touch. Rather than one partner being initiator, this position encourages both of you to give and receive stimulation. Use eye contact to communicate feelings. Be receptive and responsive to pleasuring and eroticism.

Let the decision whether to proceed to intercourse be mutual. Follow your feelings instead of doing what you think your partner expects. You can communicate with your eyes, hands, and body—it does not have to be verbal. When you rhythmically thrust your body against your partner, that is a clear communication. Continue to work toward a clear, honest, and mutually acceptable communication system whereby you feel comfortable with a range of affectionate, sensual, playful, erotic, and intercourse alternatives. Intercourse can range from a "quickie" to slow, prolonged, intense lovemaking.

Fourth Set of Exercises: Mutual Choice

Discuss whether you have fallen into any traps, such as having intercourse every time, not establishing a sensual way to enjoy each other, not negotiating a positive sexual scenario if one partner does not want intercourse or if one partner always pushes for intercourse and the other wants an alternative. If you have fallen into a trap, discuss how to develop a flexible, variable couple sexual style. Being aware of traps allows you to monitor them so they do not interfere with a vital sexual relationship. Especially be aware of the trap of inflexible male-female sexual roles and pursuer/distancer relationship roles. Satisfying sexuality, especially for married couples, involves flexibility, variability, and sharing. There is no place for "intimate coercion" in couple sexuality.

Approach this exercise with the atmosphere and clothing most conducive for an inviting sexual scenario. Begin with the male lying on top of his partner. He can move slowly down her body until his head is resting on the soft area beneath her rib cage. He puts his arms around her, with her hands free to caress his head and shoulders. This position can be particularly arousing because it positions the male where he can easily caress her genitals. There is little eye contact, but sometimes that too can be arousing. The decision whether to continue non-demand pleasuring, move on to erotic sex, or switch to intercourse should be mutual. This experience will provide an opportunity to test your signaling system because you will not have eye contact. Be aware of your needs and in tune with your partner's responses so that the sexual scenario affords you a situation in which you both feel your needs and desires have been understood and accepted.

Closing Thoughts

Comfort with non-demand pleasuring is integral to a successful sexual relationship. The knowledge that not all touching is goal-directed and intercourse-oriented enhances affection, spontaneity, playfulness, and sexual desire. A good guideline is that at least once every two months (and preferably each month) you reserve an evening for non-demand pleasuring that does not end in intercourse.

Touch is of value both inside and outside the bedroom. Being affectionate is good for your relationship and provides a positive model for your children. Perhaps the best sex education a child can have is to see his parents hugging, kissing, and caring about each other. The message to the child is that his parents feel good about themselves as a couple. Knowing that Mom and Dad love each other is reassuring for children, as is the realization that there is affection (and sexuality) after marriage.

The sexual scenarios and techniques suggested here are just a few of the many possibilities. They can be reversed and varied. It can be fun to explore different feelings, degrees of arousal, and ways of connecting. In being an intimate couple, continue to explore pleasuring positions, refine your communication system, introduce erotic scenarios and techniques, experiment with intercourse positions and scenarios, and be open to both spontaneous and planned sexual encounters.

7

Bridges: Keeping Sexual Desire Alive

Arousal and orgasm were the traditional focus of sex therapy. The Masters and Johnson research barely mentioned sexual desire. People believed the way to solve desire problems was to increase the incidence of orgasms. There is a positive relationship between sexual desire and functioning—people who enjoy sexuality, experience arousal, and achieve orgasm report higher sexual desire. However, the essence of sexual desire has little to do with orgasm. People find that hard to accept, but it is true. The four components of sexual functioning are desire, arousal, orgasm, and emotional satisfaction. Sex therapy has underemphasized desire and satisfaction and overemphasized arousal and orgasm.

Sexual desire is the most important aspect of sexuality, especially in intimate relationships. The key to enhancing desire is to understand the positive functions sexuality can play for the individual and couple. You are a sexual person from the day you are born until the day you die. Sexuality is integral to who you are as a woman or man. You are responsible for your sexuality and deserve to express your sexuality in a way that enhances your self-esteem, intimate relationship and life.

Sexuality is more than an individual behavior. Sexuality is integral to an intimate relationship. There are three primary, and one optional, functions of couple sexuality. These are 1) sex as a shared pleasure; 2) sexuality as a means to build and reinforce emotional intimacy; 3) sex as a tension-reliever to deal with the hassles and stresses of the relationship and life. The optional function is to create a baby (a great impetus for desire when it is a planned, wanted baby and an inhibitor of desire if there is fear of an unwanted pregnancy).

When sexuality goes well in a relationship it constitutes 15 to 20 percent of the relationship, its major function being to reenergize the intimate bond and generate special feelings. When sexuality is dysfunctional or nonexistent, it plays an inordinately powerful role—50 to 75 percent—drains loving feelings and causes major conflict. Sexuality, especially in its aspects of sexual desire and emotional satisfaction, can be a positive, integral element in self-esteem and your intimate relationship. Conversely, sexual problems subvert self-esteem and devitalize a relationship.

Female–Male Differences in Sexual Desire

Traditionally, women and men have learned about sexuality very differently because of the double standard in sexual matters. For women, sex has been tied to a relationship and to cooperative, interactive stimulation (a healthy learning), but not to be valued for itself (a negative learning). Sexuality has not been recognized as a positive, integral part of being a woman. Instead, female sexuality has been contingent on other aspects of life rather than being dynamic and strong in and of itself. Males have learned to value sexuality as a quality integral to masculinity (a positive learning), but as a competitive act divorced from feelings and a relationship (a negative learning). Often the trap for male sexuality is that it has not been integrated into the man's life and relationship.

During adolescence and young adulthood, the double standard favors male sexual desire. It is rare for males to report lack of desire (unless such issues as sexual orientation, fetish arousal, or sexual trauma are involved). Males experience arousal and orgasm during masturbation as well as partner sex. However, in the long run the double standard subverts the sexual desire of men. When couples stop being sexual (whether at 25, 55, or 75), in the great majority of cases

(90 percent or more) it is the man's decision. The young male's assumptions that he "should have sex with any woman, any time, and any place" and that erections come "easily, automatically, and autonomously" ultimately undercut sexual desire. He cannot meet these unrealistic performance demands as he ages. The essence of sexuality is a cooperative, pleasure-oriented, intimate sharing process.

Women report major difficulty with inhibited sexual desire. One-third of adult women have low sexual desire. For young women, fears of unwanted pregnancy and sexually transmitted diseases, concern over being labeled "promiscuous" (a sexist term used only for women), worry about personal reputation and gossip, lack of affection, and disappointment in the partner or relationship account for low desire. Traumatic sexual experiences, too, can inhibit desire—not only child sexual abuse, incest, and rape but also being exhibited to, peeped on, harassed, ridiculed, or rejected. Women have always borne the brunt of negative sexual experiences. They have maintained silence out of the fear they will not be believed and because of the cultural tendency to "blame the victim."

Warnings against sexuality (especially premarital and extramarital sexuality) have been aimed at women. The responsibility for avoiding negative sexual consequences (unwanted pregnancy, sexually transmitted diseases, sexual assault) has long been the woman's burden. The woman has not been encouraged to value sexuality for herself, only in conjunction with a relationship. Although sexuality within the context of an intimate, secure relationship is ideal, that is not the learning context for most women (or men). Sexual idealism can undermine sexual desire.

With age, there is often a reversal in female/male sexual desire. Women gain the permission to be sexually expressive; they "own" their sexuality, and aware of their conditions for satisfying sex, they develop a healthy, integrated "sexual voice." They become assertive; they make requests to increase their pleasure and arousal. Female sexual arousal becomes easier and more predictable as couples develop an intimate, interactive sexual style. Meanwhile, male arousal is changing—becoming less easy and more variable. The big difference is that male sexual response is no longer autonomous—he does not present spontaneous erections. Male sexuality becomes more like female responsiveness, so they both need pleasurable, interactive, erotic stimulation. Males who accept and enjoy flexibility and variability will not lose sexual desire. Those who long for the "good old days" are distracted by a fear of sexual performance (e.g., getting and maintaining an erection), which is the major inhibitor of male sexual desire.

Building Sexual Bridges

There are a range of sexual experiences and a variety of ways to initiate sexual activity. Being aware of "sexual bridges" to replace old patterns is crucial. These patterns were driven by novelty, illicitness, spontaneous erections, and the passionate trappings of romantic love. The media—in movies, songs and novels—present an unrealistic, fantasy version of desire as a magical and highly emotional quality. In these fictions, there is nothing conscious or intentional about sexual desire, and if it does not come passionately and overwhelmingly, something is wrong. According to the myth of sexual desire, it cannot be nurtured or enhanced; it is hot or it is not.

The approach of "bridges to sexual desire" is realistic and healthy. Romantic love, propelled by passion, is unique to a new relationship. It almost invariably fades in a year or two. If sexuality is to continue to be a shared pleasure, to nurture intimacy, to reduce tension, and to energize the relationship, healthy sources of desire and initiation have to be developed and reinforced.

What are the most important sexual bridges? Foremost is a rhythm of being sexual—sexual expression is a regular, normal, energizing element in the couple's relationship. Crucial to it is the ability of both people to feel free to initiate expression. Touching both inside and outside the bedroom is a healthy source of desire, as is awareness that not all touching has to lead to intercourse. Furthermore, sexual dates, planned or spontaneous, can add a healthy dimension to the relationship. Couples who value a range of sexual experiences—"quickies," nondemanding sex, romantic sex, sex as a break during a stressful period, sex to reaffirm caring, sex to bridge an alienated period—have a more vital sexual life than those who decree that both people need to be equally desirous each time. Fantasy is a major bridge to sexual desire for both women and men. As sexual desire often increases on vacation, going away for a weekend without children facilitates sexual activity. Use of external stimuli—sexually oriented movies, romantic music, scented candles, sexy clothing or lingerie, X-rated videos, erotic novels, mirrors—are legitimate and enhancing sexual bridges. Sex can serve as a celebration for a career success or as a consolation for a disappointment. Some couples have sex after attending a wedding as a way to acknowledge the value of their marriage. There is no limit to the bridges individuals and couples can build to facilitate sexual desire.

Many people (interestingly, men more than women) have difficulty with the concept of intentionality in sex. Our culture puts inordinate emphasis on the importance of love, spontaneity and "horniness" as the "right" reasons for desire. We are in favor of love, spontaneity and horniness, but believe there are even more healthy sources of desire. Sexuality can play a number of enhancing functions for the individual and couple. Sharing sexuality is crucial for an intimate relationship. What happens in far too many marriages is that sex is treated with benign neglect—jobs, house, kids, extended family, friends, TV, community activities take precedence. These activities are talked about and planned, whereas sex is left to the spontaneous, non-verbal realm. It is relegated to the last thing you do at night after walking the dog and watching TV. It becomes a mechanical habit, rather than a vital, pleasurable connection. If sexual desire is to remain strong, couples need to make it a priority—need to put time and energy into their sexual relationship.

One of the saddest findings is that nearly half of couples say that their sex was best premaritally. Does marriage kill sex? Is there sex after marriage? We believe sexual quality and intimacy can increase after marriage. Novelty, romanticism, and illicitness can and should be replaced by a mature emotional and sexual intimacy, by communication, by the establishment of quality sexual scenarios, by the freedom to be yourself as a sexual person and to enjoy a comfortable, functional couple sexual style. The key to sexual desire is to value sexuality, to be aware of bridges to desire, to maintain the rhythm of being sexual, to play and experiment with erotic scenarios and techniques that increase anticipation and satisfaction.

The two "poisons" for sexual desire in an intimate relationship are the emphasis on "natural, spontaneous feelings" and "romantic love." These make for great movies, novels, and songs, but they are terrible for ongoing relationships. If such fictions form the basis of sexual desire, then desire will considerably weaken within two years.

"Bridges to sexual desire" is an approach relevant to the great majority of couples. There is no "one right bridge" or scenario which works for all couples. Specific erotic scenarios and techniques help some couples but are "turn-offs" for others. One way to think about sexual bridges is to view them as the elements in a smorgasbord/buffet—you pick and choose what fits. You have the flexibility to choose what facilitates desire at a particular time and in a specific situation. Valuable bridges include planning a couple sexual date, romantic or playful touching outside the bedroom, setting a sensual mood, taking turns initiating, dropping children at a friend's and coming home to be sexual, showering before bed so you are fresh for a sexual encounter, watching an R- or X-rated video, offering a relaxing massage as a prelude to sexual stimulation, having a "quickie" after a stressful or disappointing day, using sex to celebrate a birthday or promotion or anniversary, planning a sexual date Sunday evening as a way to end the weekend.

Bob and Jeannette

Bob and Jeannette wistfully recall their fourteen-month premarital period, especially when they met for weekends (Bob lived in Boston and Jeannette in Philadelphia). Every time they got together they were sexual, their passion as strong as their anticipation. They did not need to plan sexual dates; just being together was enough to ignite the sexual spark. The five months they lived together before marriage were less sexually exciting, but they attributed that to distractions caused by marital plans and difficulties with in-laws. Shortly after marriage, arguments began about sexual frequency and initiation patterns. Jeannette complained Bob was always pushing sex, especially when they only had a short time.

Nine years later, with children ages five and two, roles were reversed. Jeannette felt Bob avoided being sexual, except for late at night. Both Bob and Jeannette looked forward to their yearly one-week trip where they left the children at the grandparents as well as their one couple weekend getaway a year. Sex was a highlight of these trips, demonstrating they still had the capacity for pleasure and passion. Jeannette wanted a healthy sexual life, but felt it needed to be at home, not just on vacations.

Unfortunately, couples seldom do "preventative marital maintenance," especially when it comes to sexuality. Sex is taken for granted and treated with benign neglect. It takes a crisis to get the couple's attention. The number one crisis is an extramarital affair. Bob had the most common type of male affair—a high opportunity-low involvement affair while on a business trip. Sex occurred after working together all day and then having three drinks; it was an intense, erotic experience. Bob planned to keep it a secret because he was both embarrassed, and afraid of Jeannette's reaction. Also, Bob wanted to leave open the opportunity to repeat the indiscretion on subsequent trips.

Bob exemplified perfectly the two adages that "affairs are easier to get into than out of" and that "affairs take more time, require more energy and are more complicated than you ever expected." The woman wanted much more than Bob bargained for. She demanded not only that he appoint her his special assistant but also that he be faithful to her and stop sleeping with Jeannette. She idealized Bob, which was flattering but scary. Bob had seen the movie *Fatal Attraction* and was afraid he had fallen into a version of it (luckily, this was an unfounded fear). He was afraid she would follow through on her threats to call Jeannette and/or file a complaint with the office manager. Bob tried unsuccessfully to finesse this situation for a month. Finally, he decided to do the courageous thing and tell Jeannette what had happened and about the dilemma he was in. Jeannette was hurt and angry, but not vindictive. Together, Bob and Jeannette met with the woman and

Bob apologized. Although there were residual negative feelings on the other woman's part, the crisis was defused.

Bob and Jeannette were left to deal with their marital issues, especially the matter of trust and the revitalization of marital sex. Rebuilding trust and sexual desire is a complex, gradual process, not the intense sexual catharsis portrayed in movies, novels, and love songs. Crucial to the process of reestablishing trust was their up-front agreement not to have affairs. If either were in a high risk situation, he/she agreed to talk to the spouse before acting out. This agreement combined with the commitment to value a couple's intimate bond is the best strategy to prevent affairs.

Rebuilding sexual desire was a complex, often confusing task. Jeannette and Bob were romanticists who wanted sex to arise spontaneously, easily and passionately—just like in the movies (and in Bob's affair). That happens early in a relationship and during extramarital affairs, but it is not the staple of an intimate relationship, especially for couples with children, careers, and a home. Couple time does not just happen, it needs to be consciously discussed and planned.

It was Jeannette who made the breakthrough. She insisted that during the week the TV stay off except for their favorite Thursday night show. This allowed her and Bob the time and space to connect so that sex was not relegated exclusively to the weekend. Jeannette embraced the concept of planning and setting aside couple time. A number of those times led to sexual encounters. Instead of Bob always being the initiator, Jeannette began initiating. Her style of initiation was quite different from Bob's. Jeannette didn't initiate verbally or in the bedroom. Jeannette's "bridge to desire" was playful/seductive touching in the kitchen, shower, or on the porch—she did not want to go into the bedroom until she felt turned on. This initiation scenario was fun and increased desire. She anticipated and valued sexuality, which in turn increased Bob's desire and arousal.

Bob was used to initiating late at night when cuddling gave him a spontaneous erection. This was not Jeannette's favorite time, but she was open to "quickies." Bob preferred she be involved in the lovemaking. Jeannette said for that she needed to be more aware and awake than she was at 11 P.M. Bob changed his initiation pattern. He put the children down for a nap or arranged for them to be watched by a teenage babysitter. He was surprised to discover Jeannette did not insist he be aroused and erect before they began. She preferred him to become aroused by her arousal and enjoyed helping him get turned on. This freed Bob to initiate teasing/playful touching to see whether it led to arousal and intercourse, and to enjoy the connection either way.

They developed "special erotic scenarios." Bob's scenario was being sexual on a warm spring or fall night after midnight (when the children and neighbors were asleep) by or on the children's jungle gym. The sense of illicitness and adventure was a powerful aphrodisiac. Jeannette's scenario was being sexual in the shower. She enjoyed sitting at the end of the tub while Bob knelt during intercourse. The pleasuring and stimulation was erotic, and washing off after intercourse was easy as could be. They might engage in their special scenario once a month or every other month, but it was exciting to know they had this to look forward to.

First Set of Exercises: Sexual Dates

You set dates to go to a movie, play bridge, make dinner reservations—what about sexual dates? Setting time for a sexual date need not be formal or overwhelming. It can be romantic and fun, and allows you to anticipate as you would a sporting event or play.

As with other exercises, we suggest taking turns. Divide the week into two parts for each of you—Saturday at 5 P.M. until Wednesday at 9 A.M. for the woman to initiate and Wednesday at 10 A.M. until Saturday at 4 P.M. for the man. This is the "Ping-Pong" system of initiation. After your partner initiates, it is your turn. If your partner did not initiate during his time, it becomes yours. The commitment is for each of you to make at least one initiation per week.

When it is your "ping," set the time, place, and sexual scenario. Do it your way, do not try to second guess your partner or compare your way to his or hers. Make the initiation as inviting as possible. Be creative in your initiations. Examples include cooking a special dinner with sex as dessert, cuddling for a half hour in front of the fire before starting genital stimulation, calling before you leave work to suggest a sexual date, surprising your spouse by joining her or him in the shower, putting on your favorite music, bringing lotion to bed and spending twenty-five minutes giving a sexual massage. Males can and do initiate creative sexual dates, contrary to the myth that romantic, seductive initiation is the woman's domain.

The woman needs to be comfortable with her ability to initiate. If sexuality is to remain a vital part of their relationship, she has to be open to creating and crossing bridges for sexual desire. Initiations could include waking her partner up in the morning (or from a nap or in the middle of the night) by sucking on his penis and putting him inside her, sharing old pictures or letters to set the mood, renting your favorite R or X-rated movie and fast-forwarding to the most erotic parts, asking your spouse to put the children to bed and meeting him in the bedroom where a scented candle is burning and you are wearing his favorite corduroy shirt, getting a babysitter and planning a two-for-breakfast hotel weekend in the city—to see art museums, eat Italian food, and have sex without worrying about interruptions.

Sex does not just spontaneously happen. It requires thought, planning, and setting aside couple time. Sexual dates are important bridges to desire.

Second Set of Exercises:
Discrepancies in Sexual Desire

If couples had to wait until both partners were equally desirous, frequency of sex would decrease by at least half. It is the norm, not the exception, for one spouse to desire and initiate sex more than the other. What poisons sexual desire is anger about non-sexual issues (which needs to be dealt with outside the bedroom) and resentment over feeling sexually pushed. Under no circumstances is it acceptable to physically force or verbally coerce your partner to engage in sex—threats have no place in a couple relationship. Sex is best when voluntary, pleasure-oriented and mutual. "Intimate coercion" leads to alienation and anger—the ensuing resentment poisons sexual desire.

What does a couple do when one wants to have intercourse and the other is not interested? This exercise will use the "yes/no" technique to deal with desire discrepancy. Our culture socializes males to always say "yes" to sex so the woman is stuck in the role of sexual gatekeeper. In fact, it is perfectly natural, normal, and healthy for males to say no to sex, and, on occasion, over 80 percent have.

In this exercise, each partner has to say at least one "no." The focus is on expanding the couple's repertoire of what is acceptable when there is a desire discrepancy. Quality of the intimate experience is more important than frequency of intercourse. Sexual intimacy is reinforced by caring about each other's feelings and sharing pleasure rather than perceiving sex as a goal-oriented power play.

This exercise requires a number of cycles rather than one structured experience. Each person will have several initiations. The initiator speaks from an awareness of what she wants—to feel desirable and attractive, unpredictability and playfulness, more orgasms, time to be alone before getting together, being valued, multiple stimulation during intercourse, affectionate touch. She asks for and initiates activities she enjoys. She is aware that her partner will say no at least once, and preferably more than once, so that they can practice at negotiating sensual and sexual alternatives. For he will not just say no, he will offer an alternative that both suits his fancy and addresses her need. For example, if she wants a whole body massage as a way of meeting her need for sensuous time before erotic contact and he is lukewarm toward a body massage, he might offer to draw a bubble bath or suggest building a fire and talking and touching in front of the fireplace. If her initiations are co-opted because he is action-oriented, she can offer a number of feeling-oriented, nonintercourse ways to intimately connect. This is the major struggle in desire discrepancy. The woman has a right to request a range of sensual and erotic interactions without her partner contending that the only real sex is intercourse. She can suggest that she manually stimulate him to orgasm, that they engage in non-genital pleasuring, that he pleasure her and she decide if she wants a mutual sexual interchange, that they have oral sex, that they share an activity (going for a walk, playing golf, going shopping) before being sexual, that he stimulate himself in her presence. He can say no to the suggestions he is not comfortable with, but needs to say "yes" to at least one of her alternatives. There are many emotional, affectionate, sensual, playful and erotic ways to connect that may or may not evolve into intercourse.

A common male trap is using sex to meet non-sexual needs. In extreme cases, males use sex like alcoholics use alcohol—to deal with emotions from anger to boredom, from excitement to emptiness, from celebration to depression. The male can learn to utilize nonsexual means to deal with nonsexual feelings. Talking about feelings is a better way to deal with sadness than having intercourse. Celebrating a merit bonus with a couple friends makes more sense than using sex as a reward.

When people talk about desire problems, the usual issue is inhibited sexual desire. However, some men use sex compulsively or to avoid dealing with issues and emotions. Hyperactive sexual desire results in an alienated relationship. Sexual bridges are meant to carry pleasure, intimacy, and tension reduction. Couple sexuality is subverted when sexual initiations carry non-sexual emotions and demands.

The man is urged to personalize his sexual invitations. Males are less likely to be distracted by nonsexual factors such as fatigue, hunger, anger, alienation, and anxiety about children. This can be a strength for sexual activity, but it can also be a source of misunderstanding and strife. The woman complains the man wants sex, not her. Making his sexual invitations and requests personal and caring is optimal.

Will the experience of saying "no" to intercourse and "yes" to sensual and erotic alternatives resolve all desire discrepancies? Of course not, but it will allow you to stay intimate friends and provide greater flexibility and degrees of freedom in expressing intimacy and sexuality.

Third Set of Exercises: Sources of Erotic Desire

There are multiple sources of sexual desire, some healthy, some less so, and some which are destructive. Healthy sources of sexual desire include (but are not limited to) sharing pleasure, feeling "horny," reinforcing intimacy, using sex as a way to connect, getting turned on by a fantasy or sexy movie, taking advantage of time away from kids, sharing loving feelings, celebrating a special date for a birthday or anniversary, enjoying the novelty of being at a hotel, making up after a disagreement, feeling erotic after sensuous caressing. Examples of unhealthy sources of sexual desire are proving something to yourself or partner, expressing anger or power, acting out a compulsive need, getting high so you can have sex, having sex after a physically abusive incident, acting out a self-destructive pattern (high-risk sex), using sex as a manipulation, and engaging in sex to run away from problems.

A persistent myth is that your partner should be the source of all sexual desire. According to this myth, if you fantasize about someone else or get turned on by seeing an attractive person, you are disloyal. In truth, fantasies and other external stimuli (movies, TV, novels, people on the street, sex pictures or magazines) are a major source of desire. Almost no one fantasizes about having intercourse in bed with her spouse in the missionary position. The essence of erotic imagery is nonsocially desirable (unacceptable) acts, people, and situations. If people were prosecuted for their sexual thoughts and fantasies, almost everyone would be in jail.

Sexual fantasies are a major bridge for desire. Sexual fantasies can be misused, especially when they are compulsive, cause shame, and/or function as a wall to shut off the partner. Generally, sexual fantasies are a healthy bridge to increase desire, involvement, and arousal.

In this exercise, each partner lists at least three and up to ten sources of eroticism and desire. We suggest sharing at least two, and keeping at least one to yourself. Sexual desire can be inhibited by sharing all and describing fantasies in detail. Sex fantasies usually work better as private fantasies rather than in attempts to play them out—the typical outcome is awkwardness and disappointment, if not disaster.

Instead of waiting for desire to "naturally" occur or expecting all desire to come from your partner, use erotic cues and fantasies to feed desire. A good example is a sexual daydream or the visual memory of an attractive person in a store. Allow that erotic image to "simmer" throughout the day so that at night it serves as a bridge for desire and sexual initiation. During the next month be aware of erotic cues and allow them to be a bridge for sexual initiation at least twice.

Fourth Set of Exercises:
Special Sexual Scenarios

People have favorite sports, music, movies. This is also true of sexual scenarios. We are not talking about "bread and butter" ways of having sex, but experiences which are "special turn-ons." One of the most interesting things about being a sex therapist is discovering the range of what individuals and couples find sexually inviting. There are the traditional romantic scenarios of dressing up, then having a gourmet dinner with wine and candles, followed by tender, loving, prolonged sex on silk sheets. There are the traditional erotic scenarios of going to a motel, watching X-rated videos, dressing in lingerie, and having sex under a ceiling mirror. For some, the key is location—being sexual in front of a blazing fire, in the shower, in an antique bed at an historic inn, on a deserted beach. For others, the key is external stimuli—erotic dancing, watching sexy videos, using lotion to cover each other's genitals, feeding the partner gourmet snacks and wine, reading erotic fantasies aloud. Many people emphasize sexual techniques—simultaneous fellatio and cunnilingus ("69"), vibrator stimulation during intercourse, mutual manual stimulation while standing in front of a mirror, taking a ten-minute wine break and resuming stimulation, engaging in one way sex to arouse the partner to total abandon, using multiple stimulation during intercourse, switching intercourse positions three times, using light bondage as a special stimulus.

Each partner initiates his/her favorite sexual scenario. A special scenario may need to be performed two or three times before it becomes a genuinely satisfying part of your couple sexual repertoire. Anticipating a special scenario is a powerful bridge for sexual desire.

Closing Thoughts

Sexuality cannot rest on its laurels. The flames of sexual desire must be nurtured and bridges to desire must be built and reinforced. Too many couples recall their best sex as new, illicit, and youthful—it is as if sex ends with intimacy, commitment , and age. What a self-defeating view! Sexuality can and should remain a vital part of a couple relationship. You can enhance the process by being aware of and maintaining bridges to sexual desire. Anticipation is the key for desire.

8

Eroticism and Arousal

We emphasize the importance of non-demand touching and the reduction of performance orientation for couples to attain sexual comfort and pleasure. However, more is required to create eroticism and arousal. The prescription for sexual satisfaction is the integration of intimacy, non-demand pleasuring, and erotic stimulation. This chapter explores the range of erotic scenarios and techniques that increase arousal.

People associate passion with a new, intense, illicit relationship in which sex is constant and driven. Just being with your partner is a turn-on. Passionate sex is powerful, special, and, unfortunately, unstable and transitory. Erotic sex connotes the "fun but dirty" approach including X-rated movies, sex shops and magazines, the singer Madonna and kinky sex. Can intimate sex be arousing and erotic as well? Is that unrealistic? We are convinced—theoretically, empirically, and in our marriage—that sex can be exciting, erotic, and satisfying in an intimate relationship. Eroticism is not reserved for pre-marital or extra-marital sex. Marital sex not only can be erotic, but eroticism is essential if you want to maintain pleasure, vitality, and sexual satisfaction.

Ideally the couple have an emotionally intimate, secure bond that has a solid foundation in non-demand pleasuring. Erotic scenarios and techniques are the ingredients that add a sense of excitement and sexual adventure.

Enhancing Eroticism and Arousal

Each couple develops a unique style of eroticism and arousal. There is no "one right way." This chapter will present a smorgasbord of choices. It is not technique alone, or even primarily, that eroticizes sex. Sexuality is enhanced by spontaneity, playfulness, and experimentation, but above all by awareness of feelings and openness to creative expression. Sexual creativity emanates from three sources: awareness of feelings, thoughts, and fantasies; a dynamic process between you and your partner that includes touching, teasing, and nonverbal cues; and openness to experimentation with a variety of scenarios and techniques. It involves acknowledging sexual feelings and desires, and taking the risk to play them out. You do not need to give a Hollywood-level performance, but you do need to share and be expressive. Eroticism and arousal need not reach for the levels of passion and lust portrayed in movies or experienced at the beginning of the relationship. What eroticism does call for are creativity, energy, letting go, and enjoying orgasmic, satisfying sex.

Routine and alienation toll the death knell for sexuality. The typical sexual scenario for "Joe and Jane Average" is sex late at night. One person, usually the male, reaches to kiss or caress and says, "Are you interested?" The scenario follows predictable five to ten minutes of foreplay, with the focus on getting her ready for intercourse; two to seven minutes of intercourse where he and sometimes she reach orgasm, a minute or two of holding and talking, and then sleep. Is there something wrong with this? Absolutely not. However, it is not the stuff of arousing, erotic sexuality. Why should sex be the last thing at night after you have finished all the important tasks of life like paying bills, putting children to sleep, cleaning, and watching the late-night comedy show? When sex is taken for granted and given a low priority, it is hard to maintain eroticism and vitality.

When people think passion, excitement, and eroticism, they focus on premarital and extra-marital affairs. Why are people willing to take emotional and sexual risks with a new person, but not with their intimate partner? They have been brainwashed by movies, songs, and sex videos that extol novelty, illicitness, spontaneity, passion, and being swept away by sexual impulses. The message is that the best sex is intense, emotional, unthinking, spontaneous, overwhelming, and "bad."

Arousing, erotic sex can and does exist in the context of a committed, intimate relationship. Intimacy and eroticism can and do complement each other. Arousing, erotic sex energizes a couple's bond and adds a special element to your intimate relationship.

Creative Sex and Multiple Stimulation

The keys to maintaining eroticism are creative sex and multiple stimulation. People can be more creative in an intimate relationship than in an affair because the commitment and communication allow the couple to take risks and let go. You do not need the disinhibition of alcohol or an affair to give you permission to be sexually creative. Creativity can include spontaneity, but the basis of creativity is thinking, fantasizing, anticipating, planning, and expressing.

There is no law that says only people having an affair meet at hotels. One of our own favorite stories begins with our opportunity to have a Sunday overnight babysitter for our children one cold February day. Barry was conducting a workshop that afternoon, so we made plans to meet at a funky, downtown hotel. Barry arrived first and signed the registration card. Emily arrived an hour later. The hotel clerk asked if Emily wanted to leave her name at the desk, reassuring her that "any name would be fine." Emily found it intriguing that the clerk assumed she was there for an affair (why would a married couple meet at a hotel on Sunday night?). Intimate couples need to reclaim their right to arousing, erotic sex. Creativity is part of sexual intimacy.

Our prescription for satisfying sex is integrating emotional intimacy, non-demand pleasuring, and erotic stimulation. Multiple stimulation is the most common form of erotic arousal. This mutual simultaneous involvement utilizes a range of erotic stimuli, allows arousal to build to high levels before you let go and abandon yourselves to passionate feelings. Special sexual scenarios and techniques can involve mixing manual and oral stimulation; playing out a master-slave scenario where the submissive partner is receiving three types of stimulation; having intercourse from the rear-entry position with the woman caressing the male's testicles while he stimulates her clitoral area; giving and receiving oral stimulation simultaneously; using fantasy to augment the intercourse experience; burning incense and listening to your favorite jazz cassette as you engage in a seductive half hour of gentle touching before switching to intense, rapid intercourse; engaging in mutual manual stimulation to orgasm as you watch an X-rated video; combining oral breast stimulation with manual clitoral stimulation while the woman fellates the male; utilizing vibrator stimulation during intercourse in the woman-on-top position while she verbalizes how turned on she feels. Multiple stimulation scenarios and techniques are a great way to practice creative sex.

Arturo and Margarita

The crisis of a discovered extramarital affair is an impetus for couples to enter marital therapy. Margarita was having an affair with a work colleague, and Arturo had short affairs when he traveled. These revelations shocked and saddened them. Friends and family members took sides and advised ending the marriage, but that was not what either Arturo or Margarita wanted.

There were a number of difficult issues that needed to be addressed for Arturo and Margarita to revitalize their marital bond. Trust and sexuality were the most important. They committed themselves to six months of couple therapy to rebuild their trust bond and sexual relationship. Through therapy, Arturo realized that sexual arousal does not exist in a vacuum. Margarita realized the importance of dealing with complex, emotionally difficult issues if loving feelings are to stay alive.

Arturo had been aroused and attracted to Margarita before marriage, but since the birth of their son, he did not think of her in an erotic manner. The thrill of high opportunity, low involvement affairs is what turned Arturo on. Margarita had been vulnerable to a colleague who found her attractive and pursued her. Margarita resented Arturo's failure to affirm her sexual desirability. She viewed herself as an adult woman, spouse, parent, competent professional, and desirable lover—and she wanted Arturo to see her that way, too.

Rebuilding emotional intimacy, strengthening the bond of trust, and non-demand pleasuring were necessary, but not sufficient. Love, trust, and communication are not enough for erotic, arousing sex. Margarita and Arturo had to value marital sex and develop erotic scenarios and techniques. This was a couple task, not the sole responsibility of either spouse. It is a joint responsibility to develop a sexual style that is erotic, arousing, and satisfying.

Arturo was enthusiastic about creating erotic scenarios. He was a visually-oriented man—he liked looking at pictures, videos, and attractive women on TV or seeing Margarita in sexy, seductive outfits were turn-ons. Although Arturo enjoyed nudity, he was more aroused by sexy clothing or seeing Margarita half-dressed. His emphasis on visual turn-ons had been off-putting to Margarita. She felt he wanted her to act as a sex object while she wanted to be seen as a desirable sexual person. Arousal and eroticism involve letting go with a sense of abandon, but not at the expense of the partner or relationship. Margarita needed to trust that Arturo's visual turn-ons included her and served as a bridge to an intimate sexual experience. A key to this process came with the realization that Arturo's desire peaked when Margarita was dressed in a sexy blouse, no bra, and black panties. His arousal in turn increased her arousal, resulting in a mutual erotic experience and a highly involving, satisfying intercourse.

Most sexual experiences are not special. Even good couples with no sexual problems are lucky if they have one or two special sexual experiences a month. Realizing erotic feelings and marital intimacy not only coexist but enhance each other was a major breakthrough for Margarita and Arturo. Experiencing eroticism while maintaining an intimate connection allowed them to "own" their sexuality. Feelings of desirability and attraction energized their marital bond.

Margarita's erotic scenarios were quite different than Arturo's. The key for her was anticipation and a slowly building eroticism that burst into a powerfully sexual intercourse. Rather than one or two scenarios,

Margarita developed four or five, with a multitude of variations. The seductive build-up could occur almost anywhere, including the bedroom, but certainly not limited to it. Margarita loved to play sexually in the car and on walks. When they left the children at his mother's, which was a one-and-a-half-hour drive, Margarita so turned Arturo on by sexually playing that they pulled off on a deserted road and had sex in the car (they joked and had fantasies about that experience for months afterward).

Margarita enjoyed the nights when Arturo took charge of the children's baths and bedtime stories because it gave her a chance to relax and read a novel (a favorite activity). She would also put on music, pour a glass of wine, and change into an outfit that could easily be slipped out of. Taking care of the kids stopped Arturo's preoccupation with work, money, and sports. He looked forward to joining Margarita for touching and music. Arturo was eager to have sex after ten minutes, but he accepted Margarita's prolonged pleasuring scenarios. She preferred building arousal to a high point before proceeding to the bedroom and intercourse. At times, she liked completing the sexual scenario in the living or family room. Arturo reacted with a combination of arousal and worry that a child would awaken. Margarita was prepared to stop if a child stirred because she did not want the children to see them being sexual. She valued the eroticism generated by sex play outside the bedroom and looked forward to the time she and Arturo would "be a couple again."

Misunderstandings about Creative Sex

The concept of creative sex is vague enough to intimidate the most knowledgeable, sophisticated couples. What creative sexual scenarios are we missing? How do we prove we are liberated? Before HIV/AIDS, there was a new, chic sexual activity introduced (usually from California or New York) every six months. This became the "in" scenario. Several years ago, the scenario was triadic sex—two women and a man. The next way to prove you were sexually free was to have anal intercourse. Six months later couples were using handcuffs and neck collars to play out dominance-submission scenes. Next came triadic sex with two men and a woman (to confront homophobia). Then there was the ultimate test of sexual freedom—being able to masturbate in front of a group to prove you were not ashamed. In our opinion, these are not indicators of creative sex, but performances to prove something to yourself or others. Sexuality is about feeling comfortable and sharing pleasure, not proving you are liberated.

The essence of creative sexuality is being aware of sensual and erotic feelings, thoughts, and fantasies and demonstrating willingness to share them with your intimate partner. Feelings and sharing are more important than scenarios and techniques. In our sexually supercharged culture, couples feel intimidated and not good enough. The essence of creative sexuality is feeling and expressing arousal as sexual play, not as a performance or competition. The problem with books like *Joy of Sex* and Madonna's *Sex* book (as well as movies and TV soaps) is that they reinforce the image that only a tiny elite are liberated.

Creative sexuality is relevant to most couples. Creative sexuality is about playing, sharing and enjoying, not "keeping up with the Joneses" or meeting a sexual criterion set by Alex Comfort, Madonna, or the McCarthys.

A key question is whether spontaneity is crucial to creative sexuality. In our opinion, spontaneity is healthy, but oversold. Once you have established a comfortable, arousing sexual scenario, it is easier to spontaneously reintroduce it. As part of the sexual mix, spontaneous encounters add a special dimension. However, at the core of creative sexuality lie erotic experiences that have become part of the couple's repertoire. These involve experimentation and verbal and nonverbal feedback. Once established, they can be spontaneously initiated and played out.

Perhaps this example will clarify the process. Jill was feeling amorous, recalling her quick but fulfilling sex with Vince two days ago. She wanted to be with Vince again, but this time desired a prolonged experience. Vince had had a busy day, but he was open to a quick, passionate intercourse. Jill told Vince their four-year-old daughter would be at a birthday party for two hours. She gave him a lingering kiss and said she wanted the whole two hours for them. As Vince drove off to do grocery shopping, his lips and penis had tingly feelings. As he walked the grocery aisles, he fantasized an erotic scenario. Vince volunteered to take his daughter to the party, which allowed Jill a respite. Vince came back to find her in a bubble bath. Although tempted by an invitation to join her, Vince found baths more relaxing than sexual. He preferred to soap Jill and take the opportunity to mix non-genital and breast stimulation. Jill shared with him how much his touching turned her on and then divulged her fantasy of making love in the family room. As Jill was putting on her favorite perfume and robe, Vince closed the shades, put the answering machine on, and chose three CDs.

Vince loved the stimulation position where he stood and Jill sprawled on the couch. Jill's favorite multiple stimulation scenario was Vince's oral breast stimulation combined with his manual clitoral stimulation while she did fellatio and he rhythmically thrust his pelvis. They switched from mutual stimulation to one-person stimulation then back to mutual. Jill was receptive to intercourse when she had already had orgasms by manual stimulation and knew that Vince was highly aroused. Her "I want you inside now" was a very stimulating invitation. For Jill and Vince, creative sex did not end with orgasm. Afterplay was an integral part of their sexual experience. Jill loved taking a nap or having Vince bring tea and fruit to bed and talking about their next couple outing.

As you listen to Jill and Vincent's sexual scenario, you might be impressed or amused. Do not worry about their way; find your own creative scenarios.

Guidelines for Erotic Exercises

What is erotic for one partner might be viewed as "kinky" or distasteful by the other. Experimentation with sexual scenarios and techniques is healthy, but within noncoercive guidelines. Experimentation should *not* be to prove anything to anyone, should not involve performance demands, and should not be manipulative. Focus on increasing eroticism and arousal rather than performance, on requests rather than demands, on honesty instead of manipulation. If you approach these exercises as mutual exploration, you will not feel pressured or intimidated.

Do not fall into the trap of feeling that you have to prove you are liberated or search vainly for the ultimate aphrodisiac. The best turn-on is an involved, aroused partner. The idea that you should find each erotic technique highly arousing is a form of sexual fascism. Discover what is erotic and arousing for you.

First Set of Exercises: Multiple Stimulation

Traditionally, stimulation has been limited to "foreplay." The man gives to the woman to get her ready for intercourse. Pleasuring involves giving and receiving stimulation, either by taking turns or mutually. Multiple stimulation extends this process to erotic stimulation in both non-intercourse and intercourse sex. Multiple stimulation is most effective when the level of arousal is moderate and building.

Let the woman take the first initiation. She can set the rhythm of pleasuring so that both partners are involved in the process of arousal. We suggest you initiate multiple stimulation in the context of non-intercourse sex, but you are encouraged to use multiple stimulation during intercourse in subsequent experiences. We provide the following smorgasbord of suggestions which you can try or modify, or you can design your own. Examples include kneeling and facing the partner, who is also kneeling, kissing, engaging in mutual manual stimulation, and requesting he use his tongue to caress her breast; she standing, he kneeling, utilizing manual vulva stimulation combined with oral breast stimulation, as she verbalizes a fantasy of his being her sexual slave; she lying on her side, he kneeling, rubbing his penis against her breast, manually stimulating her vulva, while she fantasizes about two men and two women stimulating her under a blooming tree; she lying on her back, he between her legs doing oral stimulation and simultaneously manual anal stimulation, she caressing her breasts and verbalizing how aroused she is. Continue the multiple stimulation scenario to orgasm if she desires.

When it is the man's initiative, he can introduce his multiple stimulation scenario during intercourse. Traditionally, males were only supposed to need intercourse. Whether they need it or not, most males find that multiple stimulation during intercourse increases involvement, eroticism, and arousal. In a subsequent experience, he might experiment with multiple stimulation during non-intercourse sex. Examples of multiple stimulation include from the man-on-top position, requesting that she caress his testicles while he stretches and licks her breast; from the rear-entry position, doing manual vulva stimulation as she verbalizes erotic feelings and he fantasizes; from woman-on-top, enjoying her growing arousal while playing with her breasts, she using circular thrusting; from the side-by-side position, she stroking his chest while he rubs her buttocks and they kiss each other's bodies.

Feel free to experiment with multiple stimulation scenarios and techniques; request the combination which heightens eroticism and arousal. Integrate multiple stimulation into both pleasuring and intercourse.

Second Set of Exercises: Personal Turn-ons

One of the most fascinating things about sexuality are individual differences in what people find erotic and arousing. Sex magazines and pornography try to sell people (mostly men) that "dirty and exciting" scenarios universally turn people on. They are wrong. You do not have to prove you are sexually free, sophisticated, or uninhibited. Sex is not about performance or proving anything to your partner, yourself, or anyone else. Sexuality is about touching, giving and receiving pleasure, and experiencing arousal and eroticism. Turn-ons are very individualistic.

The man takes the first initiative. Even more than multiple stimulation scenarios, there are vast differences in personal turn-ons. The following are a smorgasbord of examples which can be used by either the man or woman: Slow, mutual touching and romantic kisses followed by a rapid, intense intercourse in which both partners rush to climax; playing out a fantasy scenario (master-slave, strangers having a first sexual encounter, the sophisticated lover meets the naive, impetuous partner, the whore and virgin); making love after watching *Gone with the Wind*; waking up to your partner orally stimulating you; switching intercourse positions three times before reaching orgasm; engaging in one way sex (one person gives pleasure and orgasm without reciprocation); being sexual in the shower or right after so you are fresh for oral sex; reading a sexual fantasy aloud while the partner stimulates you following the fantasy script; using a special lotion or smell of a scented candle to heighten sensations; he giving during oral stimulation so she can have as many orgasms as she wishes; having intercourse standing up or where she is sitting on the kitchen counter; making special erotic dates for your birthday or anniversary. At a later time, the woman can design and play out her personal turn-on. Remember, personal turn-ons are not a competition; your turn-ons are usually different than your partner's. It is not a question of "right-wrong," or "kinky-vanilla." Request and share sexual scenarios and turn-ons that heighten eroticism and arousal.

Third Set of Exercises: External Turn-ons

People believe that if you are in love that is all you need to feel sexual arousal. If not, it is a sign there is something wrong with you or the relationship. The tyranny of the "shoulds," especially "love should be enough" subverts sexuality. If sex is to remain vital and erotic, feel free to utilize external turn-ons.

The woman initiates first. We will present a smorgasbord of alternatives other couples have found arousing. Each person can veto anything he finds negative, but we encourage you to be open and experimental. Examples of external turn-ons include being sexual in front of a mirror and enjoying visual feedback; using an erotic video or your favorite scene from an R-rated movie; being sexual in the guest room, living room, or family room; using vibrator stimulation as an additional source of erotic stimulation; being sexual on a deserted beach or private wooded area; having sex in a shower or bathtub; using play aids like a feather, silk sheets, mittens; being sexual in the back seat of a car as a remembrance of adolescence; using accoutrements from bondage and discipline games such as loosely tied ropes or a paddle; going to a bed-and-breakfast, funky hotel or upscale inn as a special sexual treat; using a new body lotion or scented candle; being sexual under the stars during a camping trip.

The man has his turn at initiation using external turn-ons. He is free to introduce what he wants to experiment with. Each individual and couple have their unique set of turn-ons. It is not so much that couples need external turn-ons but that external stimuli add spice to the relationship.

Fourth Set of Exercises: Creative Sexuality

Instead of taking turns with initiation, allow creative sexuality to be mutual. Each partner can contribute to an erotic scenario. This requires nonverbal and/or verbal communication. When each person's thoughts, feelings, and sexual expression flow, one's arousal enhances the other's. This is an extension of the "give to get" guideline.

Pick your favorite place to have a creative scenario (the den, bedroom, guestroom). Do not plan a scenario in detail, but be open to feelings and requests—let it flow as a mutual experience. Have favorite erotic turn-ons readily available if you decide to introduce them—lotions, a mirror, music, sexy story, beads or feathers, scented candle. During the pleasuring allow yourselves to be as free and playful as possible. Be comfortable with a multitude of positions: standing, laying, kneeling, sitting. You can have your favorite music on, dance, wrestle, play strip poker, or participate in your favorite seductive touching game. Do not set up artificial barriers between sex play and intercourse. Allow creative sexuality to flow into creative intercourse—experiment with positions, multiple stimulation, expressing feelings. Allow intercourse to be a flowing experience. Creative sexuality does not end with intercourse and orgasm. Enjoy creative afterplay, where you express, verbally and nonverbally, a range of affectionate, sensual, romantic and/or playful feelings.

Closing Thoughts

Not only is there erotic, arousing sex in an ongoing relationship, there is also a vital aspect of intimacy. Intimacy and eroticism can be successfully integrated. You owe it to yourself, your partner, and the relationship to enjoy an erotic sexuality that nurtures your intimate bond. Sexual arousal is not relegated to the young, illicit or new relationships. Eroticism and arousal are integral to intimate relationships.

9

Intercourse as a Pleasuring Experience

We have emphasized being an intimate team, feeling comfortable giving and receiving pleasure, and being aware of and responsive to erotic stimulation. These guidelines apply equally well to intercourse. All too often couples consider pleasuring as important only to set the stage. Intercourse is the "real thing." The traditional view was "sex = intercourse." Our view is pleasuring, intercourse, and afterplay are part of a continuous, flowing process. Intercourse is an integral part of the sexual experience, not an isolated activity. The best way to think about intercourse is as a special pleasuring experience.

Active Involvement

Pleasuring which is slow, tender, rhythmic, and caring allows for a natural progression into intercourse. Sexual intercourse is not a mechanical juxtaposing of two bodies; it involves the interaction of needs, feelings, and mutual pleasure. A traditional myth is that foreplay is for the female and intercourse for the male. That cheats both of them of pleasure.

The sexually aware couple enjoys the pleasuring process for itself, not just as foreplay. Pleasuring can be as enjoyable for the man as for the woman. It is not only acceptable, but preferable that both partners feel free to initiate intercourse. She can enjoy and gain as much (and sometimes more) from intercourse. Rather than assuming the role of passive recipient, the woman can initiate and be active throughout intercourse. By its very nature, intercourse involves mutuality, reciprocity, and sharing. Intercourse is most enjoyable if you are attuned to the needs, feelings, and preferences of your partner. Intercourse is the natural culmination of an involving experience of sexual sharing that begins with communication (both verbal and nonverbal) and progresses to holding, kissing and caressing, pleasuring, eroticism, arousal, intercourse and afterplay.

Intercourse Traps

The main traps couples fall into regarding intercourse are:

1. Separating pleasuring from intercourse.
2. Making intercourse a mechanical response by doing the same thing each time.
3. Making intercourse simply a penile-vaginal interchange that does not involve multiple stimulation.

To counter these traps, keep in mind the "give to get" guideline. The best way to ensure a mutual experience is to give pleasure so your partner is responsive, with each person's pleasure facilitating involvement and arousal.

Too much emphasis is placed on both partners having orgasm during intercourse. Although orgasm is important and desirable, to make it a rigid goal is a mistake. A healthier attitude is to consider orgasm during intercourse desirable only when both partners desire it. Two factors are crucial in understanding the relationship between intercourse and orgasm. First, female sexual response is more complex than male sexual response. She might be non-orgasmic, singly orgasmic, or multi-orgasmic. If the male demands his partner have one orgasm during each intercourse, he is not accepting the variability and complexity of female sexuality. He is inhibiting her, as well as himself as part of a couple, from full sexual expression. Only one in four women follow the male pattern of predictably having one orgasm during intercourse. The second factor is that there are non-intercourse methods of orgasm, including manual, oral, vibrator and rubbing stimulation during pleasuring and afterplay. These are normal, healthy sexual expressions which you are free to experience. One in three women never experience orgasm during intercourse. Female non-orgasmic response during intercourse is a normal variation, not a sexual dysfunction. Intercourse where the woman is involved although not orgasmic can be a positive experience for both partners.

Afterplay

Whether or not intercourse results in orgasm, afterplay is extremely important. Couples see orgasm as a goal, and once this goal is reached, the sexual encounter is over. This is a myth, both from a physiological and psychological viewpoint. Masters and Johnson described four phases of sexual response: excitement, plateau, orgasm, and resolution. From a physiological view, afterplay is important since it corresponds to the body's return to a less intense state (resolution). From the psychological viewpoint, an even stronger case can be made for the importance of afterplay. You have just shared an intense physical and emotional experience. Afterplay has been called "afterglow" because it is an emotional and symbolic means of showing you care about and value your partner. Pleasuring starts as a sensual experience and afterplay ends the encounter as a sensual experience. Afterplay is almost as important to an intimate relationship as pleasuring.

Positions

Satisfying sexual intercourse involves being experimental, spontaneous, and innovative. All too often couples assume there is only one proper way to engage in intercourse: male-on-top with no activity except thrusting. Within our culture, this is the preferred and most commonly employed position. However, it is a myth that male-on-top is the only normal or right position. Intercourse position is a matter of comfort, skill, and preference. Exploring a variety of positions does not mean you have to utilize esoteric skills or become acrobats or contortionists. Exploration and experimentation require only a knowledge of intercourse positions and their possible variations with an awareness of your own and your partner's needs, feelings, and desires.

Without exploration and experimentation, a couple runs the risk of continually performing stereotyped intercourse, which becomes dull and unrewarding. When sex becomes routine, it turns into a mechanical chore rather than a sharing, satisfying experience. We emphasize slow, tender, gentle, rhythmic, flowing, touching, but if each sexual experience fulfilled only these criteria, sex would also be boring and unsatisfying.

We do not want to fall into the trap of so many sex manuals by describing in great detail an endless variety of intercourse positions and variations. The mistaken message of such an approach is that you have to prove yourself a masterful technician. When intercourse becomes a gymnastic feat, it also becomes a detached, impersonal, and unfeeling experience. Instead, be aware of choices and be an active, involved participant in the sexual experience. Focus on comfort and expand your repertoire rather than perform according to a rigid criterion. Spontaneity and experimentation mean being aware of your desires and preferences and feeling free to express them.

Experimentation depends on sharing, giving feedback, and feeling comfortable. To reemphasize, sexual intercourse involves a sharing and mutuality that take into account the needs, feelings, and preferences of two people. You can expand sexual awareness by exploring intercourse positions, variations, and multiple stimulation during intercourse.

Position Variations

Popular misconceptions involve two extremes—either that man on top is the only normal position or that sexual intercourse has no limits with regard to positions. In reality, the basic intercourse positions are few in number. We will describe four positions, all of which have interesting variations and additions. Intercourse should not be used to prove something, be it sexual prowess, physical agility, or the ability to do it better than the book. Develop an intercourse style that is comfortable, functional, and satisfying.

To use the analogy of ice cream: some people prefer only vanilla; others try two or three flavors; others sample nine or ten and stay with one or two, but once a month try an exotic one; and still others try all thirty-three flavors, then make up their own. This example of individual differences is analogous to people's attitudes toward intercourse positions and variations. It is not a question of what is normal or abnormal; it is an acknowledgment of differences in style and preference.

Rob and Elaine

Is it possible to have a successful sexual relationship if intercourse is unsatisfactory? Most people, including marital therapists, would say no, but they have not met Rob and Elaine. They were a late-twenties couple who were living together, considering marriage within a year, and had worked out a number of relationship issues, especially concerning two careers.

Rob and Elaine felt attraction and arousal. They began intercourse after a month of dating, but it had not gone well. They believed it was simply a matter of time and practice. Sex problems either get better or worse—they seldom stay the same. Although their non-intercourse erotic relationship became much better, intercourse got worse. They had sex between three and five times a week, with both Elaine and Rob experiencing arousal and orgasm. However, in their once-a-month attempted intercourses, the result was intromission and thrusting, but little arousal. Rob would reach orgasm, but Elaine never did.

Elaine felt that until this problem was resolved, she was not ready to marry. Rob believed he and Elaine were a special couple and was committed to marriage. Although a private person, Rob agreed to seek couple sex therapy.

Rob did not receive adequate penile stimulation during intercourse. He complained of Elaine's passivity during intercourse in contrast to her being active during manual and oral stimulation. Elaine was frustrated because she was waiting for Rob to take the lead. He seemed indecisive and inept with intercourse. The only position they used was man-on-top, and during intercourse the only activity was Rob's thrusting. It is amazing how the learnings people have from pleasuring and erotic stimulation fall away when they switch to intercourse.

Through therapy, Elaine became aware that intercourse was not solely Rob's domain. Intercourse was a shared pleasuring activity in which she had an active role. Rob learned to ask for additional stimulation and take an involved, experimental approach during intercourse. The therapist suggested sexual exercises to break their rigid pattern and introduced the concept of intercourse as a mutual pleasuring experience. They experimented with woman-on-top and lateral coital positions, alternated who controlled thrusting, used multiple stimulation during intercourse (including breast touching, testicle stimulation, and kissing), and Elaine flexed her pubococcygeal muscle while Rob was inside her. These techniques, in addition to greater communication and the experience of intercourse as a mutual activity, increased intercourse functioning and satisfaction. At the tenth therapy session, Elaine happily announced they had set a wedding date.

Intercourse as a Natural Extension of Pleasuring

Intercourse and orgasm have been overemphasized to the detriment of naturally developing sensual and sexual responsivity. The transition from pleasuring to intercourse can be smooth and flowing. Being aware of your partner's responsivity and sharing your feelings are crucial. Arousing, erotic intercourse is a natural outcome of pleasuring. A good guideline is to engage in pleasuring that does not end in intercourse once every month or whenever you feel a need to be intimate but do not desire intercourse. It is easy to fall into the trap in which all touching becomes intercourse-oriented and you lose appreciation of the pleasuring process. Continue to enjoy non-genital sensuality and genital pleasuring. Most couples find it more erotic to make the transition to intercourse at high levels of arousal rather than in its initial stages. Intercourse is enhanced when it occurs as a choice and not as an each-and-every-time routine.

First Set of Exercises: Female-on-Top

Talk about what you have learned in non-genital touching, genital pleasuring, and other exercises you have read or tried. In particular, share feelings about the non-demand orientation, and the transition from pleasuring to eroticism and arousal. Do not fall into the trap of making intercourse a pressured, goal-oriented task.

Discuss previous experiences, if any, with the female-on-top position. Expunge the common myth that the male should always be the sexual initiator and dominant figure. Female-on-top allows the couple to experiment with a position that encourages the woman to initiate and be more active. Also, it is recommended for treating dysfunction (i.e., non-orgasmic response and ejaculatory control). At first glance, woman-on-top may seem threatening. In reality, it neither threatens nor impinges upon feelings of femininity or masculinity. It enables the woman to be active and expressive. Her arousal can in turn be arousing for her partner. It allows the man to enjoy receiving pleasure rather than having to assume the role of active, controlling partner. This can expand his awareness and enhance feelings of masculinity and sexuality.

Begin with the woman as pleasure-giver. Switch to mutual pleasuring, utilizing manual and oral stimulation. Let the movement be slow, tender, caring, and rhythmic. The transition to intercourse should be unhurried and flowing. The man can lie comfortably on the bed, with the woman straddling him by his upper thighs, with her knees bent.

Do not immediately proceed to intromission. Continue with pleasuring, allowing excitement and arousal to build. Though the male is in a passive position, he is free to actively touch and stroke his partner, to manually stimulate her vulva or move his penis around her mons and clitoral area. She initiates intromission when both feel

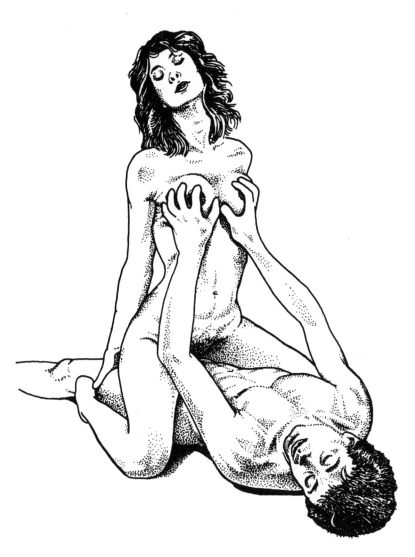

The female-on-top (female-superior) position.

aroused. An advantage of this position is that she can guide his penis into her vagina and control the depth of penetration. She can gently and unhurriedly insert the penis by sliding back on it at about a forty-five-degree angle. She can utilize whatever type of thrusting—slow up-and-down, circular, rhythmic in-and-out, or any combination thereof —she finds arousing. The man should ascertain the type of movement and speed that is comfortable and arousing for him. Experimenting and giving feedback is the best way to establish mutually enjoyable intercourse.

The man can utilize his greater freedom to caress, stroke, and fondle her body throughout intercourse. Multiple stimulation during intercourse facilitates arousal for both partners. He can stimulate her clitoral area manually. Many women find it easier to be orgasmic during intercourse with additional clitoral stimulation whether by his hands, her hands, or a vibrator. Another advantage of the female-on-top position is better ejaculatory control, so that both partners can enjoy the prolonged sexual stimulation. Be aware of and enjoy cues from eye contact and facial expressions. This is an excellent position for nonverbal and verbal communication; make the most of this opportunity.

One of the most cited disadvantages of this position is that the penis can lose containment and slip out of the vagina. We suggest experimenting with loss of penile containment. Rather than reacting with anxiety or panic (a trap for the male), use this break to engage in additional pleasuring and, when arousal is high, proceed with a second intromission. Losing penile containment does not have to be a fearful event. Rather than trying to reinsert immediately, enjoy manual or oral stimulation. When you both feel aroused and desirous of coming together, return to female-on-top with reentry being smooth and flowing. Occasional loss of containment is to be expected since the male does not control coital thrusting. The reason so many couples exclusively use the male-on-top position is that it is easiest for the male to guide intromission and maintain penile-vaginal containment. However, staying with male-on-top for security inhibits sexual expression and enjoyment.

Many couples have a difficult time with the transition from intercourse to afterplay. This transition can be comfortable and flowing rather than an abrupt stop followed by something totally different. Intercourse typically ends when the male has an orgasm. Achieving orgasm by both partners at each intercourse is a poor criterion for sexual satisfaction. Generally, at each intercourse the male will have an orgasm. However, this is not always true, specifically among older males. The woman might be non-orgasmic, singly orgasmic, or multi-orgasmic. Female sexual response is more complex and variable. She might be orgasmic during pleasuring, intercourse, or afterplay. When the male pressures his partner to have a single orgasm during intercourse, both feel demanded-upon and frustrated.

At the point the man ejaculates, the woman might have already had an orgasm (or several orgasms) or she might feel a need to be orgasmic. If she does not desire orgasm, decrease movement, stay in the female-on-top position for at least a minute, hold and touch, and share feelings. Sharing feelings is very different from clinically analyzing and rating the experience; the latter promotes resentment about being judged and results in alienation. Switch to a comfortable afterplay position where you can see and touch each other. You may want to have tissues or a towel nearby so you can wipe off the semen, or if you are comfortable with the feel of the semen on your body, leave it be.

Once you find a comfortable position, be aware of your own and your partner's resolution ("coming down") reactions. Share how you feel and what you would like—be playful, hold, stroke her hair, rub his chest, talk. Afterplay can be a good and comfortable time. Sometimes couples become re-aroused and proceed with further pleasuring or intercourse. If this happens, fine. However, do not push yourselves. Second erections are less easy to attain and second orgasms less fulfilling for the male. Afterplay is an intimate sharing experience, that is seldom oriented toward rearousal.

When the woman desires an additional or first orgasmic experience, it is important she clearly and assertively request this. The male should *never* insist *she* has to have an orgasm. This is one of our few absolutes.

We have seen the negative results of this pressure. A man partially loses his erection after ejaculation, so continued intercourse movement is irritating to his penis. Continue intercourse only if it is comfortable for the male.

There are several alternatives to help the woman reach orgasm. The man can use manual clitoral stimulation, including manual intravaginal stimulation, while at the same time orally stimulating her breasts. She can rub her pelvis against him. He can do cunnilingus. She can manually stimulate herself. He can utilize vibrator stimulation. You can combine and vary these techniques. After orgasm, the couple should continue holding and touching. Even if, and sometimes especially if, there is not orgasm for one or both partners, the afterplay experience is important. Instead of feeling unfulfilled or frustrated, afterplay offers a positive end to the sexual experience.

It is normal that some intercourse experiences will be mediocre and at least a few will be downright failures. Accept this. Do not expect each experience to be memorable. Being able to laugh about a not-so-great intercourse is a crucial ingredient in a healthy sexual relationship.

There are several variations of the female-on-top position, as there are for other intercourse positions. The woman can lie directly on top of the male, be in a semi-kneeling position, or sit up straight with her face away from him. Share feelings; discuss what you liked and did not, what to refine so you can enjoy greater pleasure. Remember, the first try at anything (recall your first experience with non-genital pleasuring) can be awkward. It takes practice and feedback to feel comfortable with intercourse and afterplay positions and techniques.

Second Set of Exercises: Male-on-Top

Male-on-top is by far the most popular intercourse position among American couples. If you use it often or exclusively, discuss what aspects are particularly enjoyable. Some commonly mentioned advantages are that it allows face-to-face interaction that facilitates verbal and nonverbal communication, and intensifies feelings of intimacy.

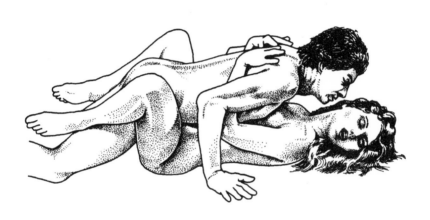

The male-on-top (male-superior) position.

Many couples find kissing during intercourse highly enjoyable. Intromission is smoothest in this position and penile containment easy to maintain. It is the best position for couples who are trying to get pregnant. The male can control thrusting, and the position allows for sustained penetration after he ejaculates. It allows deep vaginal penetration. If you are not using the male-on-top position to advantage, discuss how you might use this exercise to experiment and make intercourse mutually enjoyable.

Spend more than your usual amount of time with pleasuring. Continue pleasuring until the woman signals or initiates movement toward intercourse. Allow arousal to be high for both before beginning intercourse. Although at times minimal pleasuring followed by quick, vigorous intercourse can be erotic, one of the biggest mistakes couples make is to begin intercourse before they, but especially the female, feel sufficiently aroused.

The woman lies comfortably on her back with legs apart and knees slightly bent. She can elevate her pelvis by putting a pillow under her buttocks. The man can partially support himself by placing his knees or arms on the pillow or bed. Do not make your partner uncomfortable by requiring her to support your full body weight. When the male removes body weight, the couple is freer to share the rhythm of pelvic movement. In this exercise, he controls the type and speed of coital thrusting.

Once in the male-on-top position, do not immediately proceed to intromission. The man can run his penis around his partner's vulva and clitoral area. She can focus on the pleasurable feelings and sensations of his penis. She can take the initiative in guiding him into her vagina. He should begin coital thrusting in a slow, steady, rhythmic movement—with penetration not deeper than one and a half inches (roughly two finger joints) into the vagina—and keep the thrusting slow and rhythmic. As arousal builds, he can gradually increase the depth of penetration and rhythm of movement.

Multiple stimulation can occur throughout intercourse. A common mistake is to cease other stimulation as soon as penetration occurs. You can kiss, he can fondle her breasts, she can scratch his back, he can massage her buttocks, she can play with his chest or testicles. As she becomes aroused, do not abruptly make the thrusting rapid. Slowly increase the rhythm. Notice your reaction to rhythmic, steady thrusting. Compare that to short, rapid stroking. Does multiple stimulation throughout intercourse increase involvement and arousal?

When he ejaculates, increase the sensations by thrusting deeply into the vagina. During ejaculation most males cease movement and focus on the sensations of climax. She can be aware of his excitement during ejaculation.

After ejaculation, stay in this position for a minute or so. Look at your partner and communicate feelings about the experience you just shared. In afterplay, you might want to explore a playful mood rather than being comfortable or intimate. You could have a pillow fight, tickle each other, or play a frivolous game with your hands.

Experiment with the many position variations, including having the woman's legs fully elevated and resting on her partner's shoulders, putting a pillow under her buttocks to adjust the vaginal angle, having the woman lock her legs around his body. Man-on-top is the most common position because it has advantages for both people. It is the easiest position to maintain penile-vaginal contact. Feel free to experiment with variations in pleasuring, intercourse, and afterplay so you can fully experience and enjoy the male-on-top position.

Third Set of Exercises: Side-by-Side

Side-by-side intercourse is viewed by sophisticated couples as the most enjoyable and arousing position. However, this position does not come naturally. It takes a good deal of working together and communicating, as well as tolerating awkwardness and unsuccessful tries.

There are many variations of the side-by-side position; we will focus on the lateral coital or "scissors" position. Before beginning, agree you will use this exercise to explore and experiment and not become frustrated with yourself or your partner. A single attempt will not afford the necessary opportunity to experience its benefits. You are likely to feel self-conscious and unsure at first.

Begin with mutual pleasuring, enjoy the experience of giving and receiving pleasure simultaneously. Feel free to move and change

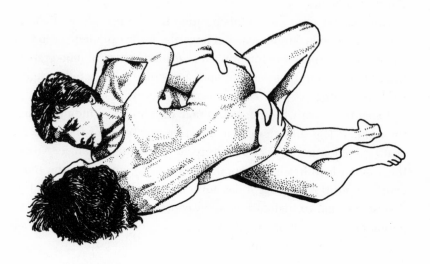

The side-by-side (lateral coital) position.

pleasuring positions. Notice some are smooth transitions (e.g., from the male stimulating the woman's breast to the couple mutually kissing and holding), while other changes punctuate the rhythm of pleasuring (e.g., after holding side by side, she disengages and moves behind him to caress his back and buttocks). Both smooth and abrupt transitions can be erotic and add variety.

The easiest way to move into the lateral coital intercourse position is from the woman-on-top position. Penile intromission is difficult (and many find impossible) from the lateral coital position. From the woman-on-top position, she, kneeling, moves slightly forward on the man's chest. As she moves forward, he helps place her extended leg behind her. She raises her other leg in a bent-knee fashion over his upper thigh (approaching his waist level). On the side where she has her leg extended toward the foot of the bed, his leg is extended parallel to her leg. She puts her head by his shoulder, and they roll to the side-by-side (lateral coital) position. We suggest not having the penis in the vagina the first time you try this. In rolling, the penis sometimes slips out. To prevent this, when the couple rolls, he can hold her buttocks so the penile-vaginal connection is more secure.

If while getting into the lateral coital position or during intercourse itself you lose penile connection, do not become upset. Simply return to the female-on-top position, and use the transition to touch and rebuild arousal.

Take advantage of the potential provided by the lateral coital position. Since you are facing each other, use eye contact and facial cues to convey pleasure. You have greater freedom of movement because you do not have to support your partner's body weight. Use that freedom to enjoy a variety of coital and touching movements and experience the sensations of whole body contact. To increase comfort, use pillows under your head or back. Place pillows on the bed so they are in easy reach after you transition to the lateral coital position.

Take advantage of access to your partner's body. From this position, more than any other, you can utilize multiple stimulation during intercourse. It is easy to shift who is directing the rhythm of coital thrusting. The partner controlling thrusting can at the same time be pleasured non-genitally and genitally. In subsequent experiences try variations, e.g., having the partner controlling the thrusting also do pleasuring. At least once, change the person directing coital thrusting. Switch rhythm or type of thrusting to be in tune with your needs. This is especially important for the woman. She can freely engage in coital thrusting to increase her level of arousal. This is an excellent position for ejaculatory control, so he can experience arousal without worrying about early ejaculation.

The couple is free to enjoy intercourse and not push for rapid orgasm. It is not mandatory that both partners achieve orgasm during intercourse. It is easier for the woman to have orgasm first because there is a good deal of pelvic and indirect clitoral stimulation and he has good ejaculatory control. If she desires further orgasms after ejaculation, he can utilize manual stimulation. Some couples enjoy doing this from the side-by-side position, others switch to a pleasuring position where the man has more freedom of movement.

One of the most harmful myths is that simultaneous orgasms are superior and vital. Setting simultaneous orgasm as a goal is a major mistake. Orgasm lasts only three to ten seconds, so striving to achieve perfect timing distracts from the mutual experience of arousal. It is frustrating if the goal of simultaneous orgasm is not achieved (which it usually is not). Accept simultaneous orgasm as enjoyable if it occurs, but do not set it as a goal. Some couples enjoy the experience of simultaneous orgasm, others feel it does not live up to its press, and others find it a disappointment.

The lateral coital position is excellent for afterplay. Continue to touch and share feelings of caring and togetherness. If you wish, you can sleep in this position.

The lateral coital position takes getting used to. To realize its benefits, you need to refine, play, and experiment. Feel free to explore variations of side-by-side intercourse.

Fourth Set of Exercises: Rear-Entry

Discuss negative reactions you might have to the rear-entry position. People confuse rear-entry intercourse with anal intercourse. Rear-entry means the positioning is altered, but the penis is in the vagina.

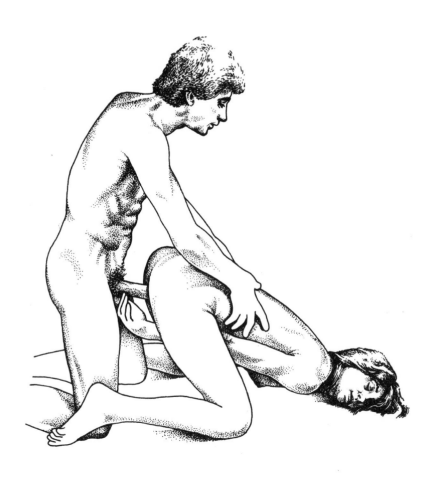

The rear-entry position for vaginal intercourse.

In anal intercourse the penis is inserted in the woman's anus. There is nothing abnormal or bad about anal intercourse. It is a variation in sexual technique that one in five couples experiment with and 5 percent use as a regular part of their lovemaking. Since HIV is most easily transmitted through anal intercourse, we strongly advise couples not to use this unless they are absolutely sure both partners are HIV negative. If you engage in anal intercourse, use a condom and/or take care to wash the penis with soap before placing it in her vagina. Vaginal infections are caused when anal intercourse is followed by vaginal intercourse without adequate hygienic measures.

A misconception about rear-entry penis-vagina intercourse is that it represents a bestial orientation, since many animals use rear-entry positioning. In reality, there is nothing primitive or animalistic about rear-entry intercourse. In Scandinavian cultures, which have a liberated sexual climate, the rear-entry position is a favorite.

Another myth is that rear-entry is a homosexual position or that people who use it are latent homosexuals. What makes an act homosexual is the sex of the partners, not the technique used. Obviously, gay men practice anal intercourse, not rear-entry penile-vaginal intercourse.

With those misconceptions aside, be aware of the advantages and discoveries available in the rear-entry position. A major advantage is that it allows the man considerable freedom in pleasuring the woman. His hands are free to caress, fondle, and stroke her body both in back and front. The sensation of his body against her buttocks is sensual and erotic. He is free to massage her mons and clitoral area during intercourse, making this an excellent position for multiple stimulation. A side-by-side variation of the rear-entry position is comfortable and minimally exerting. It is a recommended intercourse position during the later months of pregnancy.

This exercise will focus on the lateral (side) rear-entry position. Remember, the emphasis is on exploring and experiencing rather than testing your sexual prowess or performance. You need to communicate, share feelings, and experiment to discover how rear-entry intercourse can enhance your sexual relationship.

Begin with a shower or bath, being particularly aware of the buttocks as you wash them. Allow pleasure to be a free-flowing, mutual experience. Be playful—the man can run his fingers through his partner's hair, draw an imaginary circle on her body while kissing it, or tickle her feet. She might lightly fondle his chest, stomach, shoulders, and genitals as she lies behind him with her body resting against his back. Rubbing her breasts against his upper back provides enhancing sensations. When both are feeling aroused, the man positions himself behind her. As he lies next to her, he can caress and fondle her breasts, neck, stomach, buttocks, and mons.

Both partners are lying on the left side. They each bend their right legs, she extending her left leg to a comfortable position. He extends his left leg behind him and bends it slightly. When both are settled, he lifts his body high enough to guide intromission. As he guides his penis into her vagina, she can shift her body to help establish penile containment. Many women prefer to reach behind and guide intromission. Let intromission proceed slowly. If you have difficulty, do not panic or feel pressure. Remember, you are learning and exploring.

The man begins slow, rhythmic thrusting, being careful not to penetrate too deeply since in this position the vaginal canal is shorter. Deeper penetration is one advantage of the kneeling rear-entry position. The woman can guide his manual caresses over her body. She can change thrusting by moving her pelvis in harmony with his rhythm.

As intercourse continues, the man caresses her clitoral area, an action that can heighten arousal and culminate in orgasm. He should be aware whether she desires orgasm during intercourse because once the male ejaculates, he is unable to maintain penile containment. If he does ejaculate before she is orgasmic, he can use manual stimulation so she can have her first or additional orgasms. It is not mandatory that both partners experience orgasm at each encounter. Being overly orgasm-directed subverts emotional and sexual satisfaction.

The afterplay period is important in making this an integrated experience. Change positions so you have eye contact as you come down together. Discuss what you value—perhaps he enjoys the feeling of her buttocks against his genitals or touching her back during intercourse; perhaps she enjoys simultaneous manual and penile stimulation or buttock stimulation. Explore and experiment with variations of rear-entry intercourse, especially with the woman kneeling or sitting on him while he is lying on his back.

Closing Thoughts

Intercourse is a special pleasuring experience for both partners. Intercourse is best when integrated with pleasuring and afterplay. It is least pleasurable and potentially destructive when intercourse is viewed as a pass/fail performance test. Intercourse is a natural extension of the pleasuring process.

10

Special Turn-Ons

To maintain a vital, satisfying sexual relationship, stay open to playfulness and experimentation. Mechanical, stereotyped sex, even for the most loving, intimate couple, eventually results in decreased sexual satisfaction. Exploration of a variety of pleasuring scenarios and techniques enhances your sexual relationship. Sex that always occurs after eleven at night simply because you both happen to be in bed might be functional, but is unlikely to remain special.

Why do couples neglect developing special turn-ons? Some are afraid they will get into something "kinky" and become "sexually obsessed." Fear that sex will become "dirty," "sinful," or a "destructive passion" is deep in our culture. Fundamentalist ministers preach against sexual experimentation with a warning that it inevitably leads to the type of pornographic sex made infamous, until the 1990s, by New York's 42nd Street strip. The message is to stay on the straight-and-narrow or you will wind up at a sadomasochistic swingers club or worse.

An intimate couple can develop special turn-ons to enhance sexual pleasure. A steady diet of straight-and-narrow, male-on-top intercourse becomes unsatisfactory for the great majority of couples. While encouraging variety and experimentation, we suggest certain guidelines. Experimentation should not be manipulative or coercive, nor should it involve performance demands. Finding special turn-ons should be a shared, cooperative venture. The focus of sexual experimentation is pleasure, not performance; on requests and mutual choice, not coercion and demands. You do not have to prove anything to yourself or your partner. The essence of sexuality is giving and receiving pleasure-oriented touching. You are not striving to prove anything, but instead to engage in a process of discovering erotic scenarios and techniques that will enhance your intimate relationship.

Acceptance and comfort replace inhibition and anxiety. The partners should focus on increasing sexual awareness and seeing themselves as an intimate, erotic couple. Searching for the "magic turn-on" to rescue a nongiving, nonintimate relationship is doomed to failure. The basis of a satisfying sexual relationship is integrating emotional intimacy, non-demand pleasuring, and erotic stimulation. A "magic turn-on" might bring excitement for a time, but will fade quickly if there is not genuine intimacy.

Sue and Tom

Sue and Tom lived together two and a half years before marrying. This was Sue's second marriage and Tom's first. Sue had a very unhappy experience with a marriage that she had entered into at nineteen because of an unplanned pregnancy. She miscarried a month after the ceremony, yet was determined to create a successful marriage. However, it was a fatally flawed marriage. The ex-husband had no desire to be involved in a committed relationship and was physically and emotionally abusive.

Tom's relationship history was not traumatic, but it was unsatisfying. He had put his career above all else. He wanted to develop a healthier life balance with an emotionally intimate relationship and a stable, satisfying marriage and family.

Sue and Tom approached their relationship in a gradual, step-by-step manner and did not make promises they could not keep. Tom was more romantic and wanted to live together before Sue was ready. Sex was important, and they devoted the time and energy to develop a functional and satisfying sexual relationship. Sue was concerned that sex not degenerate as it had in her first marriage. Tom had an open attitude toward experimentation and was eager to find additional pleasures and turn-ons. Sue enjoyed giving Tom oral sex, which freed him to experiment with cunnilingus. Sue preferred to fellate Tom to orgasm rather than engage in mediocre intercourse. Tom had never experienced a woman who was aroused by anal stimulation as part of a multiple stimulation pattern. Sue enjoyed receiving manual anal stimulation during intercourse and cunnilingus.

They developed a special turn-on. They would stay at their friend's in-town apartment (the friend traveled a good deal on business) where they felt an adventuresomeness and freedom not present in their suburban town house. They enjoyed lounging around nude and fixing a gourmet lunch. Tom particularly liked putting food on Sue's body and sucking it off. Sue liked being sexual in the jacuzzi. This special place and the erotic turn-ons added spice to their relationship. Tom and Sue were committed to maintaining a sexual relationship that integrated affection, sensuality, playfulness, eroticism, and intercourse. They valued marital sexuality that included erotic scenarios and special turn-ons.

Guidelines for Exploring Special Turn-ons

One person's turn-on can feel silly or even anti-erotic to someone else. You do not need anyone's approval for your private, intimate sexual behavior. What you and your partner do need is an understanding about being open to and experimenting with special turn-ons. The following four exercises provide suggestions, but remain flexible enough for couples to incorporate their own preferences. Each partner can veto an exercise or part of an exercise if it is not acceptable or appealing. Experimenting with erotic turn-ons is a shared, cooperative venture. You do not need society's approval or our approval. What you do need is each other's openness, as well as respect for the other's veto power. Remember, these are requests, not demands. Sexual experimentation is voluntary and pleasure-oriented. Demands, coercion, and performance pressure have no place in sexual intimacy or erotic turn-ons.

First Set of Exercises: Oral-Genital Sex

The mouth and genitals are two of the most pleasure-giving and receptive parts of your body. Oral-genital sex is tinged with the specter of being exciting, but "dirty" or "perverse." Fellatio is the proper term (slang is "suck" or "blow-job") for the woman's oral stimulation of the man and cunnilingus (slang is "go down on" or "lick") for the man's oral stimulation of the woman. For mutual, simultaneous oral-genital stimulation, the slang term is "69." Oral sex is not only normal but one of the most intimate, pleasurable, and satisfying ways of being sexual. As with any sexual experience, there are individual differences and preferences.

Be aware of the "kinky" or "exciting but perverse" connotations fellatio and cunnilingus have in our culture. The slang terminology has a negative, and often aggressive, connotation. In X-rated movies and magazines there is an inordinate focus on fellatio, with special emphasis on domination and humiliation, specifically with the man ejaculating on his partner's face. The message is that oral sex is exciting because it is degrading—an act of lust, separate from sharing and pleasuring. What nonsense. Oral sex is pleasurable, intimate, and erotic. Oral sex is exciting and loving—an intimate sharing without connotations of dominance, humiliation, or perversion.

The best way to approach oral sex is comfortably. Begin the exercise by taking a bath or shower and washing your partner's genitals. Oral sex is facilitated by freedom from odors. Many people wash genitals before engaging in oral sex.

Some couples have no experience with oral-genital sex; others have negative or mixed experiences; some have enjoyable experiences and are interested in discovering further turn-ons. Accept your level of comfort and experience and begin experimenting from that point.

Try the giver-recipient format with the woman as pleasure-giver. The man can lie comfortably on his back, and she can use a kneeling or half-sitting position so her movements can be varied and flexible. This way she has good access to his body, especially his genitals. Begin by intermingling non-genital and genital pleasuring and engage in oral stimulation of non-genital areas. Explore various types of oral

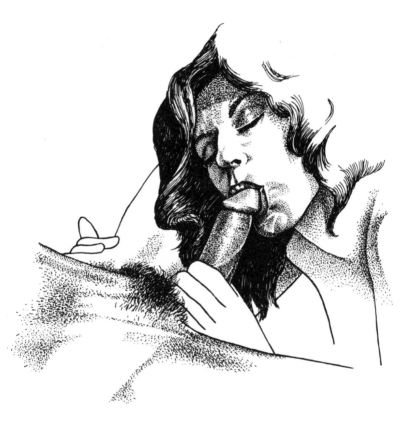

Oral-genital stimulation of male as prelude to penile-vaginal
proximity.

stimulation—kissing, gliding your tongue over his body, gentle love bites, sucking. Outline his pubic area by kissing or tongue-gliding from his navel to the inner thighs. Intermix hand stimulation with oral stimulation. You could hold and visually examine his penis while caressing and stroking it. Try tongue movements on the glans, punctuating soft, sweeping tongue motions with tongue-darting. Caress the glans with your lips while stroking the shaft with your hand. Kiss the penis from the shaft to the head. If you gently squeeze the glans, a drop of semen might come forth (a pre-ejaculatory discharge from the Cowper's gland). Semen is safe and full of protein; notice how it looks, feels, and smells. If you are comfortable with this, put a drop on your tongue and notice how it tastes.

Explore his scrotum and testicles. Look, touch, and gently kiss or suck on his testicles. If you get a pubic hair in your mouth (a fairly common occurrence with oral sex), it is nothing to be concerned about—simply remove it. If at any point you or your partner become uncomfortable or anxious, move back a step until you feel comfortable.

Put his penis in your mouth. Keep two guidelines in mind. First, to prevent a gagging response, put the penis to the side; placing the penis directly in the back of your mouth can cause gagging. The second guideline is to put your hand on the shaft so you can guide the depth and rhythm of fellatio. Some women dislike oral sex because they feel out of control; this is a way of maintaining control. Be sure to wrap your lips around your teeth because the penis is sensitive and contact with teeth can cause irritation.

With his penis in your mouth, experiment with different movements. Most women use in-and-out movements, but you might try circular movement, tongue-kissing, sucking, or gently touching his penis with your teeth. Some women find secretions from the penis to be sensuous. Be aware of and enjoy his responsiveness. Most, but not all, men find fellatio erotic. Many women find it powerfully validating to see how arousing their stimulation can be.

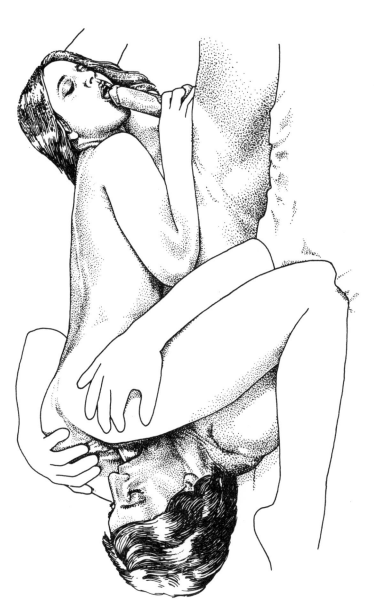

Mutual oral-genital stimulation: a special turn-on.

You have several alternatives. You can switch to intercourse, continue fellatio to orgasm, use manual stimulation to orgasm, or switch to mutual stimulation. The woman can decide how to proceed.

Each couple can choose whether or not to use oral sex to orgasm. This is not a question of normal or abnormal, right or wrong; it is a matter of personal and couple preference. Many couples enjoy fellatio as a pleasuring technique. Some enjoy continuing to orgasm, at least occasionally. If the couple chooses to be orgasmic, the man can either ejaculate into his partner's mouth or, right before ejaculation, remove the penis and ejaculate on her body or onto the bed sheet or towel. If he does ejaculate in her mouth, remember semen is safe and germ-free. Another choice, depending on personal preference, is whether to swallow the semen or spit it in a tissue or towel. The woman should do what is comfortable.

At another time, switch roles, with the man as giver and the woman as recipient. He can utilize not only his hands but his whole body by using his forearms to touch her chest, rubbing his leg against her thigh, caressing her whole body with his. Kiss, tongue-glide, and give gentle love bites on your favorite non-genital body areas. Integrate non-genital and genital touching, and intermix oral and manual stimulation. Play with kissing and oral stimulation around her inner thighs, mons, and vulva. If either of you becomes tense, move the stimulation to a more comfortable area.

When the woman feels open and receptive, begin tongue movement around her labia. Gently and tenderly explore the labia minora with your tongue and lips. Try a gentle sucking motion around her clitoris. Her vulva can be sensitive, so let your movements be tender and flowing. Be aware of the texture and sensations as you explore her clitoral area. The clitoris has as many nerve endings as the glans of the penis, but packed into an area much, much smaller. The clitoris is sensitive to touch and when arousal builds, it is covered by the clitoral hood. For most women, indirect clitoral stimulation is more comfortable and arousing than direct clitoral stimulation. Continue to intermix manual touches and caresses as you enjoy cunnilingus. Do not try to force or control her arousal; allow it to build at her rhythm and pace.

Move to the vaginal area, running your tongue around the vaginal introitus. Kiss the vagina and gently bring the vaginal folds into your mouth. Do *not* blow air directly into the vagina. While enjoying cunnilingus, continue with manual stimulation. Experiment with a variety of techniques using your tongue and lips, with kisses and sucking. As responsivity and arousal increase, let her guide you. What stimulation, where, and at what rhythm is most sexually pleasing?

Some women enjoy cunnilingus as a pleasuring technique, a way to increase arousal and lubrication. Many women are orgasmic with cunnilingus, which facilitates an involving, enjoyable intercourse. Some women find cunnilingus the best way to be sexually expressive and multi-orgasmic. There is not a "right" way to respond to oral stimulation, nor is it kinky to be orgasmic during cunnilingus. Response to cunnilingus is a matter of preference and sexual style. The advantage the woman has over the man is that being orgasmic during oral sex does not prohibit intercourse. For many women, it facilitates pleasure during intercourse. Cunnilingus is the most common technique for women to experience multi-orgasmic response (about 20 percent of women).

Share what is erotic and arousing as well as what is uncomfortable and not enjoyable. Take initiatives in guiding and making sexual requests, verbally or nonverbally. Experimenting with the rhythm and timing of oral sex is particularly important. Oral sex is most erotic when the woman is at least moderately aroused.

Some couples explore oral sex positions (standing, lying on the side, kneeling directly over the partner, the man lying between the woman's legs). A common form of oral sex is the "69" position in which you can enjoy mutual oral-genital stimulation. The sensations of giving and receiving oral stimulation simultaneously are very arousing for some, while others prefer to take turns. Be aware that as arousal builds, there is a tendency to become too rough (e.g., the male sucking too hard or the female putting her teeth on the penis). Increase the intensity and rhythm of stimulation, not the roughness.

The majority of sexually aware couples enjoy oral sex. Develop a style of oral sex that brings pleasure, eroticism, and arousal for both of you.

Second Set of Exercises: Giving to Your Partner

We have emphasized pleasuring as a cooperative, sharing experience. Yet, a special turn-on can be giving to your partner and enjoying his or her arousal, even though you are not aroused yourself. This is totally different from mechanically stimulating your partner to orgasm or placating your partner by resentfully complying with a sexual demand.

The recipient can enjoy the emotional and sexual feelings of being cared for and pleasured in a special way. He or she can let go and take in a range of sensual and erotic stimulation simply by being "selfish." The giver meanwhile receives pleasure from turning her or his partner on. The giver can enjoy feelings of power at seeing how her or his stimulation causes such obvious pleasure and arousal. Experiencing another's arousal when you are not aroused yourself can teach you a good deal about your partner's sexual response. There can be much pleasure in observing erotic flow build and seeing the partner let go. It truly can be a special turn-on for both the giver and receiver.

Be aware of your comfort and preferences. If this exercise does not appeal to you, do not allow yourself to be pressured or coerced either by your partner or this book. If this seems like a pressured dominant-submissive scenario or if one-way sex lacks allure, feel free to take a pass and move on to the next set of exercises.

Take turns being the giver. Two people do not always feel sexual at the same time. If you want to be sexual and your partner does not feel sexual, that would be a good time to try this exercise. The giver's attitude is crucial. Be open and willing to give pleasure and erotic stimulation. Your pleasure comes from your partner's emotional and sexual response. Set the rhythm of nondemand pleasuring, which evolves into giving multiple stimulation to bring your partner to high levels of excitement. Encourage your partner to let go, be selfish, and take in all the pleasure he or she can. Each person's style and preferences are different. In one pattern, the giver uses manual and oral pleasuring, stimulates in rhythm with the growing arousal, and verbalizes fantasies or uses "erotic talk." The receiver closes his or her eyes, imagines tantalizing sexual fantasies, and verbalizes erotic feelings. Allow arousal and orgasm to be uninhibited; this is your time for a special turn-on.

Be aware that one-way sex is not a competition with mutual sex.. It is a different way of experiencing each other sexually. The combination of erotic attention, along with feelings of being cared for, make this a special experience. It is not second-best to couple sex; simply different from it. There is no performance demand, just the human experience of one giving and one receiving sexual pleasure.

Third Set of Exercises: Use of Vibrators

Sexuality is one of life's most human and intimate experiences. Some are turned off by the idea of introducing a mechanical device into an intimate relationship. Yet, one of the most popular methods to enhance sexual arousal is stimulation by vibrators. The key to integrating vibrator stimulation into a couple's sexual experience is to view it not as an artificial intrusion, but as an extension of pleasuring. A vibrator can add variety to lovemaking and enhance sexual responsiveness.

Vibrators are known primarily as an adjunct to female masturbation. Some women find that vibrator stimulation enhances arousal and makes it easier to experience orgasm. Why should vibrators be relegated to women and masturbation? A vibrator can provide a variety of pleasurable sensations for both men and women.

There are different types of vibrators commercially available. We suggest a hand-held, battery-operated, two-speed model, which come with three or four rubber attachments. They are sold in drugstores or department stores as hand, face, or back massagers or can be purchased through Internet or mail-order sources.

Use the vibrator as an adjunct to touching, not as a magic toy that substitutes for partner contact. The vibrator can enhance back or body massages. Many couples use a vibrator as part of the pleasuring and arousal process, especially vibrator stimulation of the woman's genitals. Other couples use the vibrator during intercourse to increase clitoral stimulation and reach orgasm. Play with the vibrator in a way that affords comfort and enhances pleasure.

Have the vibrator available by your bed. Start with non-demand pleasuring. When you are feeling comfortable and receptive, the

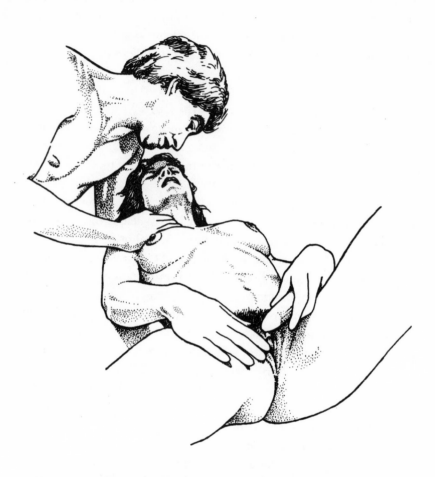

Vibrator stimulation, here being used by female in but one of many ways to enhance sexual pleasure.

woman can turn on the vibrator and press it gently against her partner's arm, leg, and chest. Try both speeds and two or three attachments. Be aware of the sensations. He can enjoy a back massage, enhanced by the vibrator. Experiment with vibrator stimulation on his inner thighs and penis. Intermix vibrator and manual stimulation. He can request and guide the type and location of stimulation.

Switch roles and allow the man to play with the vibrator on the woman's body. Get used to the variety of sensations, speeds, and attachments on non-genital areas. Take your time; be aware of and enjoy the range of sensations. Try a back or chest massage. When she feels receptive, place the vibrator on slow speed and begin on her thigh. Gradually move the vibrator until it is resting against her labia. Continue manual stimulation along with the vibrator. Then spread the labia, and gently place the vibrator around the clitoral area. The woman should relax and enjoy the flow of feelings. If at any point she becomes tense or uncomfortable, move the vibrator to another part of her body or turn it off and hold and caress her. Guide the vibrator to the most sensitive part of her genitals (usually the clitoral shaft). As she becomes receptive to the vibrator's stimulation and as her arousal builds, you can switch to the higher speed. Continue stimulation to orgasm or switch to manual, oral, or intercourse stimulation.

Experiment and play with variations of vibrator stimulation. The male could utilize the vibrator during intercourse to provide clitoral stimulation. The woman could use the vibrator herself or guide her partner in its use. He could try vibrator stimulation on his penis. Some variations might be quite pleasurable, while others are unappealing or too intense. Do not feel pressure to do something that is not comfortable. Vibrator stimulation can be a special turn-on to enhance pleasure and facilitate orgasm.

Fourth Set of Exercises:
Utilizing Sexual Fantasies

Sexual fantasies are the most common form of multiple stimulation. Both males and females use fantasies to elicit sexual desire and enhance sexual arousal. Fantasies are the most private of all sexual behaviors. People's fantasies are idiosyncratic. Sharing a fantasy is revealing a very private part of yourself. The great majority of sexual fantasies are about unusual or unacceptable people, behaviors, or situations; many are bizarre. Common fantasy themes are having sex with an unattainable partner (the boss' wife, a movie star, your spouse's best friend), being raped or forcing someone to be sexual, engaging in group sex, having a homosexual experience, being observed or observing others being sexual. What gives fantasies their erotic charge is illicitness and acting out unacceptable impulses.

It is hard to accept one's own fantasies, much less share them with your partner. Contrary to what other sex books say, we believe it is generally unwise to act out fantasies. Fantasy and behavior are separate realms. What might be extremely exciting and erotic as a fantasy can be destructive and self-defeating when acted out. Being turned on by a fantasy is not the same as wanting to actually experience the behavior. Most fantasies are best kept as fantasies; acting them out can be disappointing and place you in situations with negative and embarrassing consequences.

Is there a way to share fantasies so they are a special turn-on? We suggest doing something involving only the two of you. Be sure it is neither physically or psychologically coercive, embarrassing, or humiliating. You could verbally share and/or play out a fantasy which is exciting, exotic, unique; it does not have to be negative to be erotic. You might decide to share the fantasy verbally or to play it out. Or you might choose to pass on this exercise.

This exercise involves taking turns, since it is highly unlikely your fantasies will coincide. The man can take the first initiative. Verbally share one or two of your most erotic fantasies. If there are pictures that particularly turn you on, you could show them to her, if the turn-on involves a sexually oriented video, you could rent it and watch it together; if the turn-on involves erotic stories on the Internet, you could both be online; if the turn-on is an erotic passage in a book, you could have her read it. The majority of people find the most pleasure in verbalizing fantasies, rather than in playing them out.

If you want to play out a fantasy, it is up to you to design the scenario and guide your partner. She is aware that if at any point she feels uncomfortable or is not enjoying the experience, she has the power to say "stop." Common fantasies that couples play out involve watching the female partner do a seductive striptease, using a form of bondage and discipline whereby the partner has to trust you, lying naked in the back seat of a car or in an isolated area, being sexual on an airplane or in a high-risk situation.

When the woman initiates, she should not compete with her partner by trying to outplay or outfantasize him. She might rent an X-rated video and watch it at home, have him read from a Victorian romance novel, take sexual pictures of him or vice versa. If she desires to play out her fantasy, it is her show to be as flamboyant and erotic as she likes or as reserved and teasingly seductive as would please her. This is your personal sexual fantasy; share it and play it out your way.

Closing Thoughts

There are a variety of experiences and techniques which can be special turn-ons. Remember, the essence of creative sexuality does not lie in finding the perfect aphrodisiac or trying each new technique you read about. The essence of special turn-ons is being aware of your feelings and desires, communicating them openly, and experimenting and playing in a shared, adventuresome manner. Sexuality is most creative not when it focuses on isolated techniques, but when it involves both people in a pleasurable experience. Enjoy integrating intimacy and eroticism.

IV

Learning to Overcome Sexual Problems

11

Sexuality and Aging

A biological fact of life is that our bodies are continually changing. Developmental phases are intensely studied in children and adolescents. Much less study and research has been devoted to the aging process, especially as it affects body image and sexual functioning. Sexual changes with aging occur gradually and slowly, involve large individual differences, and are multi-causal and multi-dimensional.

Your body is continually changing in ways that affect sexual response and feelings. Little attention had been given to the effects of aging on sexual functioning until the pioneering work of Masters and Johnson. Our culture is youth-oriented and has ambivalent attitudes toward aging. These two trends, ambivalence about aging and about sexuality, have combined to make the area of sexual expression in aging (sixty and older) myth-ridden and poorly understood. Couples who desire to continue comfortable, enjoyable sexual functioning need to be aware of their bodily changes and the changes in their partners. They need to communicate and develop a positive attitude toward sexuality and aging. The more aware, comfortable, and knowledgeable they are about aging and sexuality the better. Knowledge is power.

Myths about Sex and Aging

There are myriad myths about sex and aging. A prevalent fallacy is that when a female enters menopause (typically between ages 45 and 55), her desire for sex ends. The woman who values sexual pleasure and intercourse is viewed as "oversexed." Menopause (a topic about which there are many myths) refers to changes in hormonal functioning and the cessation of the menstrual cycle and of the ability to conceive a child. The need for affection and sexual expression continues, perhaps at an even greater rate, since contraception and fear of pregnancy are no longer factors inhibiting sexual desire.

The man who does not get an immediate, strong erection or feels a lessened need to ejaculate might believe the myth he is "burnt out" sexually. Needing direct penile stimulation and taking longer to get an erection are normal, natural concomitants of aging. It is untrue that a male has only so many ejaculations and then runs out. The aging male no longer needs to ejaculate at *every* sexual opportunity. Regularity of sexual expression throughout adulthood is the best way to promote continued sexual functioning after sixty. The famous adage "use it or lose it" is based on fact.

Another myth is that sex is for the young and beautiful. According to this misconception, as you get older and lines develop around eyes, skin wrinkles, and weight increases, sexual attraction disappears and so does the need for sexual expression. When people become self-conscious, they develop a self-defeating attitude which becomes a self-fulfilling prophecy. In truth, you can enjoy sexuality in your sixties, seventies, and beyond.

A particularly confusing myth is that it is the woman who stops being sexual. In reality, in over 90 percent of couples, when sexuality ceases, it is the male's decision. He becomes frustrated with erection and ejaculation problems and decides sex is just not worth it. He feels sex is more of an embarrassment and frustration than a pleasure. It is a sad decision for men, women, and relationships.

As we age, our needs for warmth, affection, self-esteem, pleasuring, eroticism, and sexual expression continue. Being sensual and sexual is a sign of positive psychological adjustment to aging.

Changes During Aging

In the aging process there are regular, normal, and predictable changes in the body, including decreased genital vasocongestion (blood flow to the genitals). Changes that accompany aging can be incorporated into your self-image without reduction of sexual self-esteem.

You can develop a positive outlook about your sexuality and communicate it to your partner. Although the body reacts more slowly as you age, the need for sensual pleasure and sexual expression is still very much alive. Sexual responses become *different* (not worse or poorer). Whatever your age, the basic need for touching, warmth, and intimacy does not diminish; indeed, with aging, this need increases rather than lessens. Life is a balance of physical, psychological, social, and sexual components, so it makes sense that social, psychological, and sexual factors will become more important as the physical state becomes less intense. Sensual and sexual expression becomes more cooperative, interactive and intimate in the aging couple than for their young counterpart. Sexuality is an integral, positive force for the aging person and couple.

Changes during and after menopause are gradual. The walls of the vagina become thinner and less elastic, lubrication is slower and less in volume, the vagina does not expand as rapidly. If there are distressing symptoms, such as painful intercourse or uterine spasms after orgasm, the woman should consult a gynecologist or endocrinologist with expertise in hormonal management of menopause and the aging process. Hormone replacement therapy can be utilized systemically through medication or locally via an estrogen-based cream. Women should make clear to their physician that continued healthy sexual expression is important to them. Unfortunately, too many physicians believe myths about sexuality and aging or are too embarrassed to discuss sexual function and problems.

Adele and James

The most enjoyable couple Barry ever had the privilege of working with were Adele and James. Adele was sixty-four, James sixty-seven.

They had been married forty-three years and had three grown children as well as four grandchildren. They loved, respected, and trusted each other and valued their marriage. Both continued part-time employment so they had the freedom and money to pursue interests in travel, community activities, and grandchildren. They had an admirable marriage and interesting, full lives.

Their sexual relationship had always been difficult. James had a chronic problem of early ejaculation. Foreplay was relatively brief and uninventive. Although Adele enjoyed the symbolism of sexually coming together, intercourse was unrewarding for her. They were affectionate, yet the concepts of nondemand pleasuring and sensuality were totally foreign.

They were cooperative in sharing parenting before it became the vogue. They were affectionate with the kids, although not open or communicative sex educators. They kept in close contact with their adult children and grandchildren.

James and Adele regretted their poor sex life, though neither spoke of it so as not to highlight difficulties and make the spouse feel guilty. Occasionally they would read in a popular magazine or hear at a church group about the importance of communication for a sexual relationship. Although they felt closer for a week and pledged to try harder, this resolve soon fizzled out. When the media highlighted the importance of female orgasm, Adele and James decided that must be the problem. They concentrated on Adele achieving orgasm. When she became orgasmic, Adele was pleased and James felt they were on their way to a satisfying sexual relationship. However, after two months that impetus also came to a standstill.

Adele and James consulted Barry after hearing him discuss sexuality and aging in a speech about intimate marriage. Their intercourse frequency was once a month, with minimum pleasuring or sexual play. Adele and James were a committed, communicative, affectionate couple who had a solid base from which to develop an intimate, interactive sexual relationship. Therapy started by putting a prohibition on intercourse and introducing non-genital pleasuring exercises. James and Adele took to these experiences like ducks to water. When genital pleasuring was added as a natural complement, the transition from sensual to sexual was smooth. Within a month Adele was regularly orgasmic with manual and rubbing stimulation. When intercourse was reintroduced as an extension of pleasuring, Adele was aroused and lubricated. James was surprised and pleased to find he had better ejaculatory control (a bonus of aging and a comfortable sexual relationship). After three months of sex therapy, James and Adele not only had a better sexual relationship than the majority of people in their sixties, but a more intimate and erotic relationship than most couples in their twenties.

Medical Factors and Interventions

Anything that affects physical health also will affect sexual health. As people age, they are dealing with more medical problems and taking more medications, many of which have negative sexual side-effects. In addition, the body is less efficient physically. The three systems that most impact sexual functioning—hormonal, vascular, and neurological—operate less capably. In this chapter we therefore emphasize the importance of enhancing psychological, relational, and erotic factors in maintaining a healthy sexuality.

Maintaining healthy habits in terms of eating, exercising, and sleep is crucial. Eliminating smoking is important because smoking affects vascular functioning. Drinking moderately or not at all becomes important because alcohol is a depressant to the central nervous system and inhibits sexual functioning.

The Bob Dole Viagra commercials, which started in 1998, initiated a media campaign to medicalize male sexuality. While that campaign overstated the drug's promise, Viagra and similar drugs, soon to be introduced, can be a positive resource, though not as a "magic pill" to return you to your twenties. For both men and women, testosterone (the hormone most influencing sexual desire) can be valuable if medically needed, especially in the patch or injection form. For many women, estrogen supplements taken orally, in patch form, or in cream form can be of value. However, these medical resources need to be integrated into the couple's lovemaking style. Requisite for a vital, integrated sexuality as we age are intimacy, non-demand pleasuring, erotic stimulation, and positive, realistic expectations. Medical interventions need to be integrated into an aging couple's sexual style.

Sexual Gains with Aging

In discussing perceptions and feelings, older couples can emphasize the gains, not just the losses. Changes in the rate and speed of response mean that they can spend more time with pleasuring and enjoy the gradually building excitement. Slower response allows older partners to be a sensual, loving couple, because it encourages a variety of pleasuring scenarios and erotic techniques. Aging couples find that sharing intimacy and eroticism is a more fully involving, human experience than the predictable sexuality of their twenties and thirties. They can enjoy the flexibility and variability of sensual, playful, erotic, and intercourse experiences.

The exercises facilitate comfort with changes in your body. Sharing and communicating are crucial. The two major guidelines are first to support your partner as she or he strives to make positive adjustments to sexual changes; and second, to clearly and directly request and guide your partner in exploring sexual expression that includes, but is not limited by, intercourse and orgasm.

First Set of Exercises: Sensual Time

Discuss the major sexual change that comes with aging—the increase in length of time needed for arousal. An erection which was fast, automatic, and autonomous at age twenty now takes longer, needs partner stimulation, and is not completely "hard." There is a lessening in vaginal lubrication and an increase in the time to arousal and lubrication. Although your body is a less efficient sexual machine, it does provide you the opportunity to enjoy being sensual, giving, and flexible lovers.

Begin by taking a relaxing, sensuous bath or shower. As you lie together, be aware of your partner's body and of feeling emotionally close and connected. Allow touching to be sensual, warm, non-demanding, flowing. Intermix non-genital and genital pleasuring. Be aware of your own and your partner's gradually growing responsivity. Accept the sensations rather than trying to force or speed up arousal. Instead of reaching into the vagina to check on lubrication, the male partner can gently massage the woman's inner thighs, breasts, back, and shoulders. Many couples use a hypoallergenic lotion (Johnson's Baby Oil, aloe vera lotion, Astroglide, K-Y jelly) or spittle as an additional lubricant. The male should not focus stimulation on the labia, clitoris, or vagina until the woman is receptive and moderately aroused. She can meanwhile teasingly touch and caress his penis and genital area, and enjoy his slowly building erection (accept its firmness; do not compare it to the twenty-year-old athlete). Women are used to arousal coming from a giving interactive partner. Instead of the male mourning the loss of automatic, autonomous erections, he can learn to be receptive and responsive to her stimulation and arousal.

Notice your partner's building arousal. Touch in a nondemanding manner; enjoy the relaxed, sensuous atmosphere. This compares favorably to the demanding, goal-oriented atmosphere of youth. When both partners feel aroused, you can proceed to intercourse or stay with these good feelings. If you choose the latter, while holding and touching, discuss your reactions and feelings to the lengthening of sexual excitement and arousal time. If you proceed to intercourse, be sure to set aside time later to sit and discuss feelings about your receptivity-responsivity pattern. How do you feel about his less firm erection? Do you miss the quicker, heavier flow of vaginal lubrication? Can you accept your partner's slower, more involving arousal cycle? Do you enjoy the increase in sexual variability and flexibility? Integrate these changes into your feelings about yourself as a sexual person and yourselves as a sexual couple.

Second Set of Exercises: Sexual Advantages

Now that you have a sense of enhanced pleasure and understand how lengthened time for arousal can add to the sexual experience, it is time to focus on changes during intercourse. The major changes for the female are thinner and less flexible vaginal walls, decreased lubrication, and diminished intensity of orgasm. For the male, erection takes longer and requires direct penile stimulation, the need to ejaculate at each intercourse is no longer essential, the amount of semen ejaculated is decreased, ejaculatory control is easier to maintain, a waning erection requires more stimulation for re-arousal, and the erection quickly decreases after ejaculation.

Discuss changes in your body and responsiveness, and ask questions about your partner's changes. Allow the discussion to be frank, explicit, and honest. Do your experiences follow the information presented or do they differ? Remember, each person and couple is unique. The female partner might want to know how the man feels about stimulating her as she becomes aroused and about sensations of vaginal containment. How does he feel about her orgasmic response? Does she enjoy helping him get an erection? How does she feel about changes in erectile ease and predictability? Can she feel when he ejaculates? He might want to inquire about her reaction when he does not ejaculate. With aging, female sexual response is easier and more predictable than male. How do each of you feel about this? It is a reversal of your sexual socialization and experiences—can you welcome and enjoy it?

It is important to accept natural body changes, to support your partner in making positive adjustments, to view sexuality in a broad-based manner, and to view intercourse as part of the sexual repertoire rather than as the main (or only) act. Be open to experiences that are available as a result of the aging process—specifically the man's ability to better control ejaculation and the woman's ability to maintain arousal. Sexual arousal becomes a more interactive, cooperative experience. Enjoy gradual, mutual whole-body sensual and sexual arousal.

Use pleasuring techniques—non-genital touching, genital touching, oral stimulation, non-demand positions, whole-body contact, multiple stimulation—which facilitate mutual arousal. Enjoy the gradual build-up, and take pleasure in observing your partner's excitement. Be supportive, warm, giving, and loving. Enjoy a sexuality that is more intimate.

Instead of demanding that the man get an erection (such a demand increases pressure, which increases anxiety and decreases arousal), the woman can use a variety of manual and oral penile stimulation techniques. As his arousal builds, so will his erection. The male can deal sensitively with the slowness of lubrication, accepting that she may be subjectively aroused but her physiological responses are more extended. Do not raise her anxiety, which would decrease arousal and lubrication, but continue with sensual and sexual touching, which naturally leads to heightened arousal. Experiment with K-Y jelly, a hypoallergenic lotion, or your spittle for additional lubrication. Self-consciousness is anti-erotic. Enjoy involvement in the pleasuring process and the erotic flow.

Before initiating intercourse, be sure both of you are receptive. Do not pressure yourself or your partner. Intercourse is not a performance test. Even if the man's erection is not completely hard, be aware that when he becomes aroused, it will be firm enough for penetration. The woman can guide intromission. She can caress his penis and actively facilitate insertion. She can also direct coital thrusting and experience maximum feelings and sensations. During intercourse, continue slow, tender, rhythmic movements. Enjoy the warmth and erotic feelings. Instead of focusing solely on penis-vagina contact, engage in multiple stimulation—touching, fantasizing, caressing. Multiple stimulation during intercourse is an effective arousal technique for old and young alike. You can enjoy the entire experience and not fall into the youthful trap of expecting and demanding rapid genital release. The woman can enjoy being orgasmic (whether before, during, or after intercourse) and notice it is a whole-body sensation rather than an intense, focused genital experience. As the male ejaculates, he can enjoy the feelings that have developed throughout pleasuring and intercourse. Focus on the sensual and sexual feelings throughout your body, and accept the less commanding genital sensations. Celebrate the heightened sharing, flexibility, and variability. Sexuality and aging facilitate an integrated, broad-based sexual experience. It may be less physically intense, but it is more intimate and fulfilling.

To complete the experience, bask in the afterplay phase. While holding and touching, discuss how pleasuring, erotic stimulation, and intercourse can continue as a vital part of your intimate relationship.

Third Set of Exercises: Erection and Ejaculation

This exercise focuses on making a positive adjustment to one of the more threatening aspects of the aging process—the less predictable erection and lessened need for ejaculation. During youth, erections were easy, automatic, and autonomous, and ejaculation accompanied each intercourse. Even if young men are fatigued, drink too much, are not aroused, or become stressed or ill, they consider the lack of erection or ejaculation to be a failure.

Men do not have the knowledge or experience to understand and accept changes in erections and ejaculatory demand. The sexually functional woman accepts a built-in variability in her arousal and orgasm experiences. She experiences orgasm as integral to her sexuality, but learns to accept and enjoy nonorgasmic experiences and not consider them as negative or a failure. However, she is used to her partner ejaculating every time they have sex and overreacts when he does not. She can and should support him in making a positive adjustment to more variable, flexible patterns of erection and ejaculation.

What the man learns to accept is that it takes longer and requires more direct penile stimulation to obtain an erection. Arousal and erection are dependent on psychological awareness, couple intimacy, and partner stimulation and arousal. He can have pleasurable intercourse, but will not feel the need to culminate in orgasm each time.

The man has to adopt the approach his partner has practiced for the past thirty years. He has to be affectionate, sensual, playful and erotic, and see those qualities as being important and valuable in themselves. Erection and ejaculation happen when the flesh is able, but their absence is not indicative of a lack of sexual interest or pleasure. Erection, intercourse, and ejaculation are not the sole factors in sexuality for the older male as they were in his twenties.

This exercise should be done a day or two after an ejaculation when the man is feeling little or no ejaculatory demand. Enjoy pleasuring, arousal, and intercourse. Both partners focus on making the interaction arousing, prolonging stimulation, introducing the penis into the vagina under the woman's guidance, and enjoying the total sexual experience. Be aware, though, there is no demand or desire to ejaculate. Your penis is responsive to stimulation and you enjoy arousal and erection. There is pleasure on intromission and during intercourse. If your partner is aroused and desires orgasm, you both can enjoy her sexual satisfaction, whether during intercourse or with manual, oral, or rubbing stimulation.

Experiment with ways to make this a positive sexual experience. The man might want to cease intercourse and be manually stimulated, to roll over and hold her, to ask her to give him a whole-body massage using a lotion, or to sit, touch, and talk. Make this a pleasurable experience in which you enjoy a broad range of sensual and sexual activities, including intercourse. The trap for the male is to feel the experience is worthless if he does not ejaculate—and to push himself to ejaculate. The trap for the female is to commiserate with her partner about his "failure" or push him to ejaculate in order to prove that she is still sexually desirable. This is self-defeating. A woman can have a positive experience without orgasm; so can the man.

Your sexual relationship will be enhanced if you both feel positive about non-ejaculatory experiences. Ejaculating only when there is a desire for orgasm, and accepting it is normal for the male not to ejaculate will do much to maintain enjoyment of sexuality and intercourse into your sixties, seventies, and beyond. A reality of sexuality and aging is role reversal—female arousal becomes easier and more predictable than male arousal. Enjoy the changes, accept them instead of fighting them.

Are the sexual techniques the man used to help his partner be orgasmic acceptable and enjoyable for him? Feel free to experiment with scenarios and techniques to enjoy a broad-based, flexible sexuality that does not center solely on erection, intercourse, and ejaculation.

Fourth Set of Exercises: A Special Time

Set aside two hours or more. You may want to include a glass of wine, one mixed drink, or an herbal tea. You could put on music, view an erotic video, recite your favorite poems, look at special pictures, or read X-rated stories.

Take a sensuous bath or shower and lie in bed nude. The male can begin by caressing his partner's body and, while touching, describe how it looks and feels. If at any point the woman feels uncomfortable, she can interrupt and check what he meant or is feeling. She should not focus on what she has lost, but on here-and-now feelings about her body image, desirability, and sexuality. She should trust her partner's perceptions and feelings and listen to what he says about the lovely, sensual parts of her body. She should be aware of and accept bodily changes and a new body image. There is more to sexual self-esteem than a young firm breast that has grown heavier. It is still your breast and a good part of you. Accept bodily changes gracefully; this facilitates viewing yourself as an attractive, sexual woman. So does the male's expression of loving support both verbally and by touch. The fact that the woman knows he enjoys touching her enhances sexual intimacy.

Switch roles and let the woman caress the male's body while being aware of and commenting on changes. Be open and honest in acknowledging differences in his bodily responses while showing him support, affection, and caring. Accept changes in his body tone, the wrinkles on his skin, the gray hair—he is not in training to be a sexual athlete or a movie model. He is aware of differences and relishes the positive experience of prolonged pleasuring and sensual feelings. Erections take longer to achieve and there is greater need for active stimulation and shared pleasure. Arousal is maintained by give-and-take stimulation. Rather than the aging process taking away sexual expression, it is building and reinforcing sensual, whole-body feelings. Sexuality is an involved, cooperative sharing in a giving, intimate relationship.

Intercourse can follow an extended period of pleasuring. Give and receive multiple stimulation before and during intercourse to enhance involvement, eroticism, and arousal.

After the sexual encounter, stay with feelings of closeness. Afterplay could involve sharing a drink, a talk, or a pillow fight. Then return to touching. The male will not get a second erection, nor will he have a desire for a second ejaculation. The female is aware of a lessened need for arousal and orgasm, but the need for touching and affection remain strong. Allow your second coming together to be a sensuous, whole-body experience that can overcome fears or negative feelings about your attractiveness and sexual desirability.

Closing Thoughts

The aging years constitute one of the most significant times in life for enjoying feelings of caring, sensuality, and sexual expression. Sexuality over sixty is normal and healthy. The best way to ensure effective sexual functioning is to stay actively involved in sensual and sexual pleasuring and not to make performance demands. Enjoy and appreciate your body, your partner's body, and couple intimacy. The integration of intimacy, non-demand pleasuring, and erotic stimulation reaches fruition with aging. Allow sexuality to be a positive part of your relationship into your sixties, seventies, and beyond.

12

Enhancing Your Sexual Relationship

We have emphasized the importance of communication, experimentation, and intimacy. You are in the process of changing sexual attitudes, behaviors, and feelings, and of developing a comfortable and satisfying sexual style. This chapter will explore how to enhance your sexual relationship.

If companies put as little time and energy into their business as couples put into their marriage, we would have a bankrupt country. The chief guideline in maintaining and enhancing sexual intimacy is to put a priority on couple time. An intimate relationship needs to be nurtured and valued. If your sexual relationship is taken for granted, it stagnates, becomes boring and routine, and can degenerate into dysfunction or dissatisfaction. Love that is not growing is dying. Your intimate relationship needs consistent attention and caring. Sexuality serves to energize the marital bond and generate the special feeling of marriage. When sexuality goes well it is a small (15–20 percent) but integral component in marital satisfaction. However, when sexuality is dysfunctional, fraught with conflict, or nonexistent, it plays a powerful (50–75 percent) negative role and saps the relationship of vitality and good feelings. Sexual problems are like a cancer, destroying the intimate bond between partners.

There is a joke that you can spot people having affairs as opposed to married couples. The former are attentive, caring, and affectionate people who are aware of each other. Married couples do not talk intimately, seldom show affection, and do not attend to each other's emotional needs.

A major reason couples enter marital therapy is the crisis over the discovery of an extramarital affair. If people stopped having affairs, it would cause a recession for the practices of marriage therapists. A prime reason for affairs (along with ample opportunity) is the feeling that individual emotional and sexual needs are not being met in the marriage. When Barry counsels a couple, he urges them to avoid the blame/guilt trap and instead to focus on the meaning of the affair in the context of their marriage. Why did the affair happen at this time? What needs were not being attended to in the person's life and marriage? Is there a commitment to revitalize the marital bond? How can trust and intimacy be rebuilt? If the couple successfully deals with the affair, it will increase commitment to a quality, satisfying, stable marriage.

If you believe the spate of self-help books, every marriage will experience an affair or major crisis. It is the "chic" thing to say among "sophisticated" couples. Marriages do experience transitions and the person and the relationship need to change if marital sex is to remain vital and satisfying. However, affairs and marital crises are not the preferred—and certainly not the most psychologically efficient—way to facilitate change. Although one-third to one-half of marriages do experience an affair by one or both spouses, prevention is optimal (and less emotionally and financially draining).

Suzanne and Kevin

Suzanne and Kevin are a committed, intimate couple. On their twenty-fifth wedding anniversary, instead of the formal party, which is often just a ritual, they took a month's vacation. The first two weeks were spent together and the last two with their adult children (and new grandchild).

Kevin and Suzanne reviewed their married life, its highs and lows, its successful and painful transitions. Their courtship had been very romantic. They had dated fourteen months, and started intercourse four months into the relationship. The sex was exciting and added to their loving feelings, but, in retrospect, they admit that the quality was poor. Kevin was intense, goal-oriented, and ejaculated rapidly. Suzanne was not orgasmic until eight months into their marriage. She enjoyed sex, but was reticent to voice her sexual preferences and make requests of Kevin.

They very much enjoyed Suzanne's first pregnancy and together attended prepared-childbirth classes. Kevin was present at the birth of their daughter. The adjustment to being parents is a major one for almost all couples, but it was easier for Suzanne and Kevin becuase they shared parental responsibilities. It was during the second pregnancy that their sexual relationship blossomed. They felt they were in love before they married, but realized that romantic love was a myth—a delightful, but temporary state. Developing a mature, intimate relationship meant accepting the spouse as an individual with strengths and weaknesses while still respecting and caring for each other. Mature intimacy is based on the individual being his or her own person within a genuine bond as a couple, rather than coming together out of loneliness, dependency, or need for acceptance. After five years of marriage, Kevin and Suzanne were independent individuals, had developed their style as a couple, and were attuned to each other's sexual feelings and preferences. The relationship grew more intimate as they shared experiences and feelings.

All marriages experience transitions and difficult periods. For Kevin and Suzanne the seventh through ninth years were troublesome. The children were at demanding ages, requiring large amounts of time and psychological energy. Kevin and Suzanne enjoyed their home but were short on financial resources, which created a constant stress. All vacations were family-oriented, so there was little time for each other (it was not until their tenth wedding anniversary that they learned the importance of trips without the children). Kevin was in a workaholic phase, trying to push his career ahead. Suzanne resented his preoccupation with work, but seldom voiced her feelings. Through these mediocre and stressful years, their respect and commitment remained solid. This was a relatively joyless period and, as might be expected, sexual encounters were less frequent and less pleasurable. Yet sex continued to provide positive reinforcement and to reduce tension.

A church-sponsored marriage-encounter weekend reversed this stagnant pattern. Kevin and Suzanne did not like the pro-family values proselytizing or the dialogue technique, but they did value the time and opportunity to honestly share concerns, dissatisfactions, and requests for change. Kevin realized he had to do better at balancing his roles as parent, husband, and worker. Suzanne realized she was falling into the role of the resentful, dissatisfied housewife, and had to broaden her horizons. Both became aware of the need to be spontaneous and playful sexually. Sex should not be relegated to late night hours after they had done all the important things like paying bills, cleaning the kitchen, and watching TV.

Upon reflection, Suzanne and Kevin realized they had experienced a pattern of alternating cycles of relatively calm years with years of change and transition. They made an agreement that every six months they would discuss how their lives were going and consider future plans. Probably the best decision they made was to take a risk and move to an area where they had long dreamed of living. They recall with extreme fondness making love the first night in their new house, on a mattress on the floor, surrounded by boxes.

One predictable source of marital stress is parenting adolescents. Kevin and Suzanne were fortunate in that their children were good students, did not abuse alcohol or drugs, and were socially and athletically active. They worried about a number of things, not the least of which was their children's sexual activity. They tried to educate them in matters of sexuality, but found it no easy task. The adolescents were reluctant to talk or ask questions. They were more likely to bait their parents and make fun of how "hung-up" and old-fashioned they were. Suzanne and Kevin were consistent in encouraging their adolescents to have good relationships and enjoy being affectionate, but not to have intercourse while in high school. They advised their children to wait until they were in a meaningful relationship and then to proceed safely, with contraceptives, in the face of STDs/HIV.

Contrary to popular myth, rather than the "empty nest" syndrome, Kevin and Suzanne experienced a rebirth in their marital and sexual relationship when their children left home. They enjoyed the freedom from day-to-day parenting concerns. They relished the increased time they could spend on individual and couple activities (including greater sexual flexibility). Both enjoyed being with their adult children and particularly their new grandchild, but the most important bond in a family is the husband-wife bond. This is true throughout child-rearing years, and even truer once children leave home and you are a "couple again."

Suzanne and Kevin were wise to realize they could not rest on their laurels. The next twenty-five years would be different as they entered new life stages. There would be further transitions in their lives and marriage. They are committed to discussing and planning career and life changes. Kevin hoped to do more supervisory work and take a month's vacation yearly, accepting the fact that Suzanne's career, which is heating up, will allow her to accompany him only two of the four weeks. Very seldom are people's lives in perfect synch, but a healthy couple accepts and supports each other's personal growth while maintaining "coupleness." They looked forward to "nooners" as well as being sexual in the morning and early evening. They planned to set aside a time once a month to engage in sensual and genital pleasuring with a prohibition on intercourse. Suzanne was particularly excited about initiating creative erotic scenarios.

There are lots of juggling balls to balance in people's lives—personal identity, being a couple, parenting, careers, house-upkeep, friends and extended family, community and political interests, religious and intellectual pursuits, and sports and leisure. Kevin and Suzanne had done an admirable job of balancing without letting the sexual "ball" drop. Sexuality is a positive, integral part of their lives and marriage. Although there is no longer a procreative function, sexuality is still a shared pleasure, a means of reinforcing intimacy, and a tension-reducer.

A good sexual relationship may not solve individual and couple problems, but having a satisfying sex life enhances and energizes your intimate bond. The following exercises focus on stratagems to increase intimacy and satisfaction rather than on sexual techniques.

These guidelines offer a way to enhance your intimate relationship and foster psychological growth. An intimate relationship requires time, energy, respect, trust, and caring. A good marriage can survive crises, but does not require crises for growth.

First Set of Exercises: Couple Time

The prime guideline for an intimate relationship is to set aside couple time. Couple time can be anything from a five-minute talk over a cup of tea to a forty-five minute walk after dinner, to setting aside an afternoon for lunch and sex, to a weekend away without the children. The essence of couple time is sharing hopes, perceptions, plans, worries, and feelings rather than discussing practical day-to-day matters, children, jobs, or money. It can, and usually does, involve affectionate touch and may or may not include being playful or sexual. Couple time acknowledges and reinforces the value of your intimate relationship.

Each partner will have the opportunity to initiate an activity. What element of couple time would be of particular value? Would you like a romantic lunch on Saturday afternoon as a prelude to a sexual date? Go into your bedroom in the early evening, start with a back rub, and gradually build to intercourse? Bathe together once a week and discuss intimate feelings while basking in the warmth of a bubble bath? Sit over a drink on the porch, hold hands, and talk? Have your feet rubbed or hair combed and move to playful sex?

What do you want to share? For some people, the important thing is to be listened to—that is enough. For others, discussing thoughts, hopes, or fears is important to feeling close and loving. Some couples find great value in talking about a problem and brainstorming alternatives. For others, revealing dreams or fantasies is a way to relate intimately. What thoughts, feelings, problems, or issues would you like to discuss and share? Now is the time.

How do you communicate whether you want to be affectionate and share sensual pleasure or whether you are interested in arousal and orgasm? A major reason couples do not set aside time is that they are unsure of hidden sexual agendas and worry that it could turn into a tense scene.

Couple time has value apart from sexual expression. Couple time might include touching and sensuality 50 to 75 percent of the time, and involve sexual arousal and intercourse perhaps 20 to 40 percent of the time. Both people can feel free to initiate, and both are free to say no and offer an alternative. You can develop a clear and comfortable communication system whether couple time will include touching, sensuality, playfulness, eroticism and/or intercourse.

Be aware of the value of your intimate relationship. What can you do to enhance emotional and sexual intimacy?

Second Set of Exercises: A Couple Weekend

A weekend away. It takes time, money, planning, and babysitting or housing children with another family. Is it worth all that trouble? It is one of the wisest investments you can make. Can you afford not to do it? Whether it is a weekend or a week, recharging your batteries as a couple has real value. In our complex, hectic world with individual, work, community, and family responsibilities, treating yourself to a time away at least once a year is important, if not crucial.

Instead of one person being totally responsible for this activity, divide the tasks. One could get reservations and the other arrange for childcare. Where to go—the beach, mountains, the city for plays and shopping, home with the phone off the hook and no projects? Do you want to do something physically active—sail, hike, play golf? Or something calmer—go for long walks, eat at a gourmet restaurant, search for antiques? Much of the weekend time is spent as a couple, but we strongly encourage you to also set aside individual time.

The best marriage is between two responsible individuals who choose to share their lives in an intimate way. Healthy relationships balance individual and couple needs. Enjoy intimacy and sexuality on your couple weekend.

Third Set of Exercises:
Being Sexually Adventurous

When people think of exotic or erotic sexual scenarios, they usually think of youthful couples, extramarital affairs, or the jet set, not of themselves. Give yourselves permission to be sexually adventurous and erotic. We are not advocating an activity that would cause discomfort, violate your value system, or be considered "kinky." Certainly, you should not force or coerce your partner to participate in a sexual scenario which would make him or her uncomfortable or that he or she would not enjoy. Sexually adventurous experiences are most satisfying when they are freely and mutually entered into. You have probably read about, thought about, or fantasized sexual scenarios you want to try but which you have not given yourself permission to discuss or explore.

Let us offer a list of suggestions, some of which we are comfortable with ourselves and some of which we are not. Each individual has his or her own sexual values and comfort level. How do you feel about these scenarios? Making love outdoors—on a beach, in the woods, in your back yard; renting an X-rated video; trying anal intercourse; using a super-deluxe vibrator; going to your office when no one is there and having sex on your desk (or in the boss' office); acting out a master–slave or bondage fantasy; having dinner in the nude and having each other for dessert; having intercourse in the shower; having sex during a mock fight.

What are your fantasies or desires? To guard against the experience being negative or causing recrimination, consider the following guidelines: Only participate in what you choose; if you become uncomfortable, you have a veto power and your partner agrees to stop. This exercise is for exploration and pleasure, not to prove you are sexually liberated. If you feel coerced, stop the experience. This is a shared co-operative venture. You can choose to pass on this exercise.

Each person gets one initiation (do it at a different time rather than both the same day). Tell your partner what you would like to try so you are sure he or she is open to it. In playing out the exercise, let go and be involved; self-consciousness is anti-erotic. Make this a special erotic experience. Do not try to second-guess your partner. Partners can express their feelings and alter the experience if they want. Each partner gets to initiate a sexually adventurous scenario.

After the experience, discuss how you felt. Is this something you would like to continue on special occasions? Do you want it to be a regular part of your sexual life? Was it a disappointment? If so, do you want to try a different sexually adventurous scenario?

Anticipating special erotic experiences is a way to keep sexual desire vital. Even if they occur only once a year, like making love outdoors, they are adventurous additions to your intimate relationship.

Fourth Set of Exercises: Do It Yourself

We have structured sexual exercises as guidelines to provide an opportunity for you to experiment, discover, and share what is comfortable, pleasurable, and erotic. The process of gaining awareness, exploration, and sharing feedback is continuous; it need not end with these exercises. This is the foundation—you can continue to grow and enhance your relationship, especially by being spontaneous, playful, and erotic.

In this exercise, do your own thing: be experimental and creative in a way that is particularly you. You might focus your creativity on pleasuring fully clothed or spending fifteen minutes in a totally sensuous encounter. You might focus your creativity on intercourse—trying a position with the woman sitting and the male kneeling so that he can massage her breasts and clitoris during intercourse, or with the couple in a sitting position (female lowers herself on her partner who is seated on the bed, chair or thick carpet), or with both partners standing or switching positions at least twice during intercourse. You might focus your creativity on the afterplay experience: You could hold each other while keeping your eyes closed, sit nude and express your feelings through intense eye contact for five minutes, have a playful pillow fight, share sensitive material that will help your partner better understand you or try a position that is comfortable enough to sleep in. Do your own thing to enhance intimacy and sexuality.

Closing Thoughts

These exercises present a set of flexible guidelines and suggestions. Decide what is beneficial for your intimate relationship. How can you enhance sensuality and sexuality? Be open to intimate feelings and share them. Explore and experiment. Be clear and direct in your feedback and requests. Nurture and enhance your intimate sexual relationship.

13

You As a Sexual Person

You are a sexual person from the day you are born until the day you die. A healthy attitude includes seeing sex as a good aspect of life; maintaining sexuality as a positive, integral part of your personality; and expressing sexuality in a manner that enhances your life and intimate relationship. Men and women are sexual in similar and complementary ways that enhance their bond as respectful, trusting partners in an intimate relationship.

This perspective on contemporary intimate relationships differs drastically from the traditional Victorian or double-standard views that most adults have grown up with. Negative learnings about sexuality, especially that sex is "exciting but dirty" and that men and women are very different sexually, inhibit sexual desire and functioning. Sexuality is a way to express your human need for touching, sharing, and pleasuring. This need is equally valid for women and men.

You can increase awareness of and comfort with sexuality. This is not a demand to feel sexual and perform at any time, in any situation, with any partner. That is the sexual pressure traditionally placed on the male. It is as antihuman a view of male sexuality as the traditional female imperative to not be sexual at any time, in any situation, or with any person other than her husband—and even then not be carried away with passion. You can learn to be comfortable and accepting of yourself as a sexual person. It is your choice to be sexual at a time and in a manner where you can genuinely celebrate healthy sexual expression.

How do people learn about sexuality? There are many sources, but a prime one is through touch. The touching you receive as an infant from your mother and father is important; so is your own touching to explore your body. Before the age of six months, most children discover the positive sensations of touching their genitals. Was playing with your penis or vulva accepted by the parent as normal and healthy or were your hands slapped and told: "No, that's dirty"? Our approach is not intended to blame parents for adult sexual problems. Your parents acted according to what they knew; it has only been in recent years that sex educators and researchers have advocated acceptance of childhood sexual curiosity and exploration. We believe you as an adult can undo negative learnings and build a healthy sexual awareness and comfort.

The child's touching himself is likely to include both non-genital and genital touch. The child is experiencing positive feelings, not genitally oriented sexual arousal. That child has an important lesson to teach adults. Sensuality is the basis of sexuality. The child feels he is entitled to the warm, comfortable feelings of sensual touch. Genital exploration and stimulation are a natural extension of sensuous touch.

Masters and Johnson, the pioneer sex researchers, point out that you can neither will nor force sexual response. No one, including us, and no book, including this one, can teach you how to become sexually aroused and have an orgasm. The potential for sexual response is natural. What you can learn is awareness of sensual and sexual stimuli, how to nurture sexual desire, the importance of clear and direct communication, and active involvement in giving and receiving pleasure. Be open to your sexuality, not inhibited by the "roadblocks" which interfere with healthy sexual expression. The most common roadblocks are anticipatory anxiety, performance anxiety, trying to impress your partner, goal-oriented sex, forcing sexual response when you are not turned on, using sex as a weapon in an argument or power struggle, using sex in a manipulative manner, doing something sexually that you are not comfortable with or that violates your values. Sex is not a performance to prove something to yourself or your partner, nor is it a spectator sport. Performance orientation inhibits desire, pleasure, and satisfaction. Sexual awareness is facilitated by being open and receptive to affectionate, sensual, playful, erotic, and intercourse touch. The essence of sexuality is giving and receiving pleasurable touch.

Susan

Susan was a good example of a person who inhibited her sexual desire. She was thirty-two, divorced, and had custody of her two children. She had received little sex education other than the jokes and stories of friends. As an adolescent, Susan was attractive and popular, but felt pressured by boyfriends. Although she enjoyed the attention, affection, and excitement of touching, she felt ambivalent and held back. This pattern is typical of the dating experiences of adolescent and young adult women. The woman fears being taken advantage of. She is concerned about pregnancy, sexually transmitted diseases, and being labeled "promiscuous" (a term used only for women).

Susan's most powerful negative learning came from the double standard. The young man assumed the role of initiating and pushing sex. He was supposed to be sexually knowledgeable and experienced. This put Susan in the position of fending off sexual advances and not saying what she wanted or making requests (she was afraid of leading her boyfriend on). When she was expressive (making sounds and/or engaging in pelvic thrusting), her partner told her that was not the "right" thing to do. Susan became embarrassed and altered her sexual responsivity, which diminished her arousal.

Susan became pregnant at eighteen and entered into a fatally flawed marriage. She felt out of control of her life, and blamed sex as the culprit. Four years later, after a sexual relationship that focused on her husband's needs rather than hers and resulted in another unplanned pregnancy, he left her for another woman.

Susan was suffering from low self-esteem, depression, and difficulties coping as a single parent (neither the ex-husband nor her parents provided financial resources). Luckily, she had the support of a women's group and entered a career training program. At thirty-two Susan was professionally competent, financially secure, and responsible for herself. Unfortunately, she had not transferred these attitudes and behaviors to her sexual life. After dating for two years, she decided that she was merely repeating adolescent experiences, and it was not worth it. She did have male friends, but had not had a sexual relationship in four years. When a friendship with a man became romantic, Susan panicked.

Susan consulted a female psychologist with a specialty in sexuality issues. The therapist emphasized that Susan had a right to choose whether or not to be sexual. If she chose to be sexual, it should add to her life, not just meet the man's needs. She was urged to consult a gynecologist and use an effective contraceptive (she chose the birth control pill). Rather than striving to be orgasmic, Susan focused first on being comfortable with her body and self-image. She engaged in a self-exploration program which improved her sexual self-esteem. Susan utilized sexual fantasies to enhance self-stimulation, enjoying images of men servicing her as if she were a powerful queen. Soon Susan viewed herself as an attractive woman and was able to be assertive and tell her partner what she needed practically, emotionally, and sexually. For the first time, Susan was looking forward to being an involved, active sexual person.

Sexual Choices

Whether a man or woman, you are entitled to make choices about sexuality, including choosing to be nonsexual. You can enjoy sex without having to prove anything to yourself or your partner. You do not have to apologize for or defend your choices. You deserve sexual comfort, pleasure, and satisfaction.

Sexual desire means "you want to." You can nurture sexual thoughts, images, and fantasies. Feeling that you deserve to enjoy sex and can anticipate its pleasures is crucial for sexual desire. Use fantasies to anticipate and rehearse a sexual interaction. Fantasies are a mental turn-on which facilitate desire and receptivity to touching and arousal.

The cultural stereotype is that women need encouragement to be sexual, but that men do not. According to tradition, the man needs nothing emotionally or sexually; he could have sex with any woman, at any time, in any situation. What a terribly demanding (and demeaning) myth! It is especially burdensome for the man with inhibited sexual desire. Male desire problems are a secret he tells no one, especially male friends, for fear of ridicule. It would be easier to admit to an erection problem than to admit there is low or no sexual interest. The male does not even tell his wife or partner what he is feeling; he avoids sex by working too hard, drinking too much, or having another headache.

Men need to be more accepting, less critical, and less demanding of themselves sexually. Young males experience anxiety, guilt, and confusion about sex, but rarely do they have problems with desire or arousal. This is because males learn to masturbate early and frequently view sex as a way of confirming their masculinity, and also because males use sexually explicit fantasies. Male sexuality is tied to youth, illicitness, and automatic, autonomous erections. For a middle-aged man, these sources of sexual desire are not as strong, and men often fall into the trap of viewing themselves as "over the hill."

The man can develop a new, healthier way of understanding himself as a sexual person. He needs to rid himself of the pressure to be a " stud" who can induce sexual desire and produce an erection at will. As he ages, he is less a sexual athlete, but more an involved lover. Which is more important—that he gets an erection without needing the woman's touch or that he enjoys the give-and-take of sexual sharing? As he ages, sexual desire and arousal become a shared, cooperative experience. This can be of great advantage for the man and his sexual relationship.

A man can feel masculine and sexual as he ages, as long as he accepts bodily changes and adopts healthy attitudes. Of special importance is to value shared pleasure, rather than feel he has to perform for his partner. Does the man give himself permission not to feel turned on at a specific occasion? Is he entitled to say no to sex? He is a sexual person, not a sexual machine.

Alex

Alex is a fifty-one-year-old married man who has experienced inhibited sexual desire for the past four years. Alex talks wistfully of experiences as a young man when sex was the major thing on his mind and he had erections whenever he saw a woman. He had several premarital partners and married Darcy when he was twenty-seven. Alex reported a lessening of sexual desire at thirty, after three years of marriage and two children. In his thirties and forties Alex had sex once or twice a week. When out of town, he would occasionally go to a prostitute or massage parlor (practicing safe sex) because he felt that is what "real men" did. He considered his sex life average and moderately satisfying, but gave it a low priority.

About four years ago, Alex's oldest son began living with his girlfriend. Alex had ambivalent feelings. He liked the woman and was glad his son was in a stable relationship, yet he was worried about couples "living together" rather than marrying. Alex envied his son's sexual relationship because he himself felt "used up" and less sexual. Rather than discussing this with Darcy, male friends, or a therapist, Alex decided to remedy the problem by having an affair with a younger woman as a "tonic." This affair provided sexual excitement, but caused major problems. Alex felt used by the woman in many ways, including financially. When the affair was discovered by a friend and reported to Darcy, it provoked a strained and embarrassing six-month period. For the next three years, sexual desire disappeared from Alex's life. He would occasionally have sex, at Darcy's initiation, but had difficulty maintaining an erection. This frustrated and depressed Alex, and increased his tendency to avoid sex. He would occasionally masturbate, especially after a poor experience with Darcy, to reassure himself that physiologically everything was functional.

Alex came to therapy after reading an article about inhibited sexual desire. His first question was: "Am I normal?" Alex was seen individually and then with Darcy. The therapist helped Alex clarify what he valued about sexuality and the benefits of revitalizing marital sexuality. Alex had a negative self-esteem as a middle-aged man, did not anticipate sex, and believed the myth that the best sex was "youthful and illicit"—like his son's. He had lost his erectile confidence.

Self-defeating attitudes and the desire to return to youthful sex are major causes of inhibited sexual desire in middle-aged men. These causes have to be confronted and replaced with healthy attitudes and new strategies, including non-demand pleasuring, erotic stimulation, and developing a cooperative, give-and-take intimate relationship. This puts new life into the sexual relationship and allows men to adopt an attitude of sexual challenge rather than mourning the loss of youthful sexual vigor. Sexuality becomes pleasure-oriented, intimate and interactive, although less automatic and predictable. As Alex's interest and desire returned, his erectile comfort and confidence also returned. If it had not, Viagra or a similar drug could serve as an additional resource to rebuild his comfort and confidence with erections. In the past few years, physicians have used Viagra as a "magic pill" for desire, erection, and almost anything else sexual. It would not have helped Alex, however; not in and of itself. Males have to make attitudinal, psychological, and sexual changes if Viagra is to be successfully integrated into the workings of their sexuality. Alex valued Darcy's sexuality and their give-and-take stimulation. They did not have that in their twenties, so in many ways sex in their fifties was more involving and better quality. Their experiences inoculated Alex and Darcy from sexual problems in their sixties and seventies.

The focus of the exercises is to become aware of what you personally value about sexuality and to identify ways to increase desire. Identify blocks and inhibitions to sexual desire that need to be confronted and challenged. The exercises are learning and exploring experiences, not performance tasks. You cannot fail at an exercise. Be aware of what you can celebrate about yourself as a sexual person.

First Set of Exercises: Sexual Self-Esteem
Set aside at least a half-hour when you have privacy and are not distracted or worried. Give yourself permission to focus on the sensitive topic of your sexual self-esteem.

You might want to sit in a comfortable chair, have relaxing music in the background, and keep at hand a pen and notebook to jot notes to yourself. Start by doing a personal historical inventory.

Where did you first hear about sexuality—from parents, friends, religious education, siblings, on the street, through reading? Was sex supposed to be good and exciting or was it evil and fearful? What were your parents like as a sexual couple? Were they affectionate with you and your siblings? What do you remember about touching and exploring your body as a child—was it okay or were you told it was bad? What about sexual play with children in your neighborhood or with siblings or cousins? When did you first stimulate your genitals—did it feel good or were you anxious and guilty? When did you carry self-exploration through to masturbation? Did you enjoy being orgasmic? For men, what was your reaction to your first nocturnal emission (wet dream)? For women, what was your reaction to your first menstruation—was it a transition into womanhood or a source of embarrassment?

How old were you when you started dating? Did you think of yourself as attractive and a good person to go out with? Were initial dating experiences good for your self-esteem or did they cause unhappiness and feelings of rejection? Did you enjoy being affectionate—holding hands, kissing, hugging? Was touching and sexuality an easygoing part of the relationship to be experienced and explored, or a double-standard battleground where the male was trying to prove something and the female was pressured and stressed? When was the first time you were sexually aroused with a partner? What about first orgasm with another person—did you feel good about sexual expression? First intercourse is an important experience for both men and women; it is often a disappointment—what was it like for you?

By age twenty-five, 95 percent of people recall at least one sexual experience which they felt bad about, confused by, guilty over, or traumatized by. What were your most negative experiences? In addition to the trauma of incest, rape, and child sexual abuse, other negative experiences include guilt over masturbation or fantasies, having an unwanted pregnancy or sexually transmitted disease, being sexually humiliated or rejected, being peeped on, exposed to, or sexually harassed. Do these negative experiences still cause guilt or trauma or have you integrated and accepted them so they do not affect your sexual self-esteem?

What are your attitudes and feelings about being a sexual adult? Do you feel good about your body? Are you responsible for yourself sexually? Do you use effective contraception? Roughly, four in ten people contract a sexually transmitted disease (herpes, chlamydia, genital warts, gonorrhea, syphilis, crabs). Do you think of this as a medical problem to have diagnosed and treated, or do you see it as a punishment for sex and thus put yourself down as a "bad" person? Have you had an unplanned, unwanted pregnancy (roughly, one of three women have)? How did you handle this dilemma? Has it left any psychological scars?

What have you learned about yourself and choosing a healthy relationship? What aspects of a partner do you most value? What makes for a good sexual relationship? What was your best sexual experience? Did you "own" the experience—feel you desired and enjoyed it? How can you now improve sexual desire, comfort, and pleasure in your life?

As you complete this self-guided sexual history, be aware of the positive and negative elements of your sexual development. All of us have a sexual history. We have never met a person who did not have bad experiences, negative learnings, or regrets. People are responsible for their sexuality and, with increased awareness and understanding, can have a healthy sexual life in the present and future. You owe it to yourself to develop a positive sexual self-esteem.

Second Set of Exercises: Body Image

Our culture is obsessed by physical attractiveness and youth. Look at the ads in magazines and on TV—youthful, stylishly dressed, attractive men and women selling everything from soap to cars. It is as if to consider yourself attractive, you have to look like a star.

Positive body image is integral to sexual desire. You can accept yourself as an attractive person without having a perfect body. We are opposed to people undergoing plastic surgery every two years. We are equally opposed to the person who no longer attends to personal hygiene, does not shave, gains sixty pounds, and wears rumpled clothing. Seeing yourself as a sexual person involves accepting your body and emphasizing components that increase attractiveness.

Set aside at least an hour of private time. Lay out three clothing outfits—a formal one, an informal one, and one you consider sexy. If possible, have access to a full-length mirror. Wash and groom yourself in a manner you find attractive. Put on your favorite formal outfit and look in the mirror. What do you like best about your appearance? Do you see yourself as an attractive adult who takes care of him- or herself? Think of the compliments you have received when you were dressed formally; instead of dismissing them, realize you are an attractive person.

Put on your sexy outfit. It could be a dressy ensemble, a swimsuit, an unbuttoned shirt and pants, or a favorite nightgown or pajamas. As you look in the mirror, you might try changing your hairstyle, facial expression, or stance and posture. Enjoy different aspects of your body image. Do not be embarrassed or inhibited about being expressive in front of a mirror. Give yourself permission to experience different dimensions of yourself and body image. See yourself as a desirable, attractive person.

Switch to your informal outfit. You do not need to be dressed formally or seductively to have an attractive self-image. Some people like a clean-cut, well-pressed image; others prefer a low-key, informal image; still others like to look distinctive and unique. What is your style preference? Give yourself permission to promote positive changes in your image, especially in your view of yourself as a sexual person.

Be aware of the images, clothes, and attitudes which add to your feeling of being an attractive, sexual person. Focus on these at least twice a week for the next month as you reinforce an image of yourself as a sexually attractive and desirable person.

Third Set of Exercises: Sexual Fantasies

If people were to know about your sexual fantasies, they would be shocked and you would be embarrassed—true or false? The socially desirable answer is "false," but the reality is "true." More than any other element of sexuality, fantasies are your private domain. Even more than masturbation, fantasy is a private experience. Why? Fantasies by their very nature involve socially nonacceptable thoughts, images, people and situations. We do not fantasize about having intercourse in bed with our spouse. We fantasize about sex with a movie star, our best friend's spouse, an exotic person, a stranger, someone of the same sex, a relative. We fantasize less about intercourse, more about oral sex, being tied up, raping or being coerced, performing simultaneously with four people who admire our sexual prowess, simultaneously engaging in oral and anal sex, being sexual with an animal, being in a threesome with our spouse looking on in horror or fascination. In fantasy we do not have sex in our bedroom, but on a beautiful beach, in the office with everyone looking on in envy or disgust, in front of a thirty-foot fireplace, on a movie set. People's fantasies would be embarrassing and humiliating if advertised on TV. The source of sexual arousal lies in this "forbidden fruit" aspect of fantasy.

The essence of sexual fantasies is their unacceptable, strange nature—this is what makes fantasies an erotic turn-on. Fantasy and behavior are very separate realms. People feel anxious, guilty, or fearful of acting out fantasies. Fantasies are not meant to be experienced in reality, but to be relished as harmless, exciting, sexually arousing images. Fantasies serve as a bridge to initiate sex and heighten arousal. Fantasies are problematic when the person obsesses on one fantasy, experiencing high levels of arousal with concomitant high levels of anxiety, guilt, or shame.

Give yourself permission to focus on a range of fantasies and images without judging and putting yourself down because they are "dirty," "weird" or "lustful." Enjoy the fantasies and images, allow yourself to feel sexy and "horny." People pair fantasies with self-stimulation. You can use your imagination or material like *Playboy, Forum, My Secret Garden,* or a book, Internet material, magazine, or video you find erotic. You might be turned on by visual material, stories, or mental images—use what works for you. Go with the fantasy; let it carry you rather than you direct it. Sexual fantasies have a life of their own with a strong emotional, irrational component. As you experiment with sexual fantasies, do not become obsessed with just one. The mind is your private X-rated cinema—enjoy the variety; it is free. Learn to enjoy fantasies for what they are: a positive part of sexuality which increase desire and arousal.

Fourth Set of Exercises: Erotic Scenarios

One of the nicest things about being a child was your birthday when everything was designed to please you. Seldom does that happen as an adult. We suggest couples designate "caring days," when their likes and emotional needs are given special attention. Almost never is this done in the sexual arena. This exercise gives you permission to experience your favorite erotic scenario.

Plan a day to enhance sexual desire. You might start with breakfast-in-bed, take a walk in the woods, have a midday nap, listen to your favorite music, enjoy your partner's affection and caring, be pleasantly surprised by an inexpensive gift, bottle of wine or full body massage, go to a movie, have dinner at a new restaurant, delight in a long, luxurious bath. Where does sex fit? It could be in the morning, before or after your nap, in the early evening, or at the end of this special day.

What would be a pleasurable or erotic scenario? It could involve being stroked and caressed for as long as you desire, experimenting with an oral sex position you have read about but were too bashful to try, being stroked in front of a mirror where you enjoy visual as well as tactile stimulation. What about playing sexually for ten minutes, taking a bath, then being submissive to your partner's every desire, perhaps using two intercourse positions you have not tried for ages (sitting facing each other, rear entry, standing up, the woman sitting on the man)? Does she enjoy multiple stimulation—him orally stimulating her breast, with one hand stimulating her clitoral area and the other stimulating her anal area? Some males (and females) like active, abandoned sex where she "attacks" him and strokes his penis hard, sucks intensely during fellatio as he rapidly thrusts his pelvis, then engages in intercourse involving deep, fast, rhythmic thrusting. Other men (and women) like a sexual scenario which is slow and tender with lots of intimate, loving verbal exchange. Choose your erotic scenario; play with it, enjoy it. You do not have to limit the scenario to one special day; enjoy eroticism in your ongoing sexual relationship.

Closing Thoughts

Sexual desire is not something you either have or do not. It is a multi-dimensional set of attitudes, behaviors, and feelings which reflect you as a sexual person. Remember, sex is a good thing in life and sexuality is an integral part of your personality. You are responsible for your sexuality. Express sexuality so it enhances your life and intimate relationship.

14

Becoming a Sexual Couple

The keys to individual sexuality are feeling comfortable as a sexual person and assuming responsibility for a sexuality that enhances your life and intimate relationship. Your partner can neither bestow nor force sexual desire on you. You alone are responsible for your sexuality and sexual desire.

Our culture is dominated by fantasy images of sexuality. Romantic love, instant intimacy, the magic of sex! Being swept away by romantic love is a seductive myth. "Romantic love" seldom lasts even to marriage. The images and concepts presented by the media (novels, songs, movies) are counter-productive for people trying to renew or maintain a vital sexual bond.

We propose a more realistic approach to developing and maintaining sexual desire in your relationship. This approach will help you attain and maintain a sense of yourselves as an intimate sexual couple. Sex is a healthy sharing experience between two people who are aware, comfortable, and responsible. An emotionally and sexually intimate relationship is not easy to attain (or maintain), but once achieved, it is very worthwhile and satisfying.

Talking Sex

How to begin? If you are like most couples, you have had both exciting and disappointing sexual experiences. Other than joking or perhaps blaming, you have not honestly and openly shared sexual attitudes, feelings, and experiences. You justify this by saying that you do not want to remove the mystique from your sexual relationship. It is true that you can talk and analyze a sexual relationship to death, making sex so clinical and self-conscious that it lacks all semblance of fun. However, most couples err on the other end of the continuum, by not discussing sexual feelings, preferences, or intimacy at all.

Most couples do not have a comfortable sexual language. "Proper" terms such as *penis, vagina,* and *intercourse* seem formal and lifeless, whereas "slang" terms such as *prick, pussy,* and *fuck* have an angry, derogatory ring to them. An alternative is to develop your own sexual language. What would you like to call your penis or vagina? What is a comfortable word or phrase for intercourse? Do "making love," "getting together," "having sex" work for you? Develop a sexual language which allows you to communicate comfortably and clearly.

Couples need to be comfortable sitting and talking clothed if they are to be comfortable in the nude having intercourse. Talking, kissing, and touching in affectionate, nondemanding ways provide a solid base for your sexual relationship. Holding hands or walking with an arm around your partner's waist is an important element of intimacy. Sexuality encompasses more than genitals, intercourse and orgasm. The base of sexuality is sensuality. To build sexual desire is to develop an enjoyable, sensuous, intimate way of being with each other.

Accepting yourself as a sexual person enhances your attractiveness. Being an aware, responsible sexual partner facilitates becoming a desirous, satisfied sexual couple.

Alice and Brent

Alice and Brent had a satisfying sexual relationship, but allowed it to dissipate by taking sex for granted and not nurturing intimacy. It surprised and embarrassed them to have a sexual dysfunction because they prided themselves on being sexually liberated and sophisticated. They had lived together for eight months before marriage, when Alice had been twenty-seven and Brent twenty-six. They fondly recalled staying up half the night making love in their efficiency apartment. In the intervening thirteen years they had in many ways grown and matured; they had bought a townhouse with a lake view, had two children they enjoyed, held reasonably well-paid jobs (although Brent felt stuck in his career), and took pride in their personal achievements.

After two years of marriage their sexual life became unsatisfactory, and in the past three years it had become dysfunctional. They had unsuccessfully attempted to reverse this course by a number of poorly thought out, half-hearted efforts. These included buying *The Joy of Sex* and trying one of the "pickles," going to a "sex motel" with X-rated movies and a vibrating bed, having a group sex experience at an ocean resort (this was particularly risky in terms of STDs/HIV, although they used condoms). Brent and Alice even had affairs to see if that would make a difference. The affairs proved to be more complex and disruptive than either of them had bargained for. Two generalizations can be made about affairs: they are easier to get into than out of, and they take more time and psychological energy than expected. Affairs are not a healthy way to solve a couple's sex problem, although many people with sexual problems have an affair.

As often happens when couples experience relationship difficulties, the problem is reflected in a sexual dysfunction or dissatisfaction. Alice and Brent sought sex therapy several years later than would have been advisable. A good guideline is that if a sexual problem lasts for more than six months, it will probably not spontaneously remit, and you should seriously consider consulting a therapist.

In assessing the problem, the most important factor that emerged was the erosive state of Brent and Alice's marital bond. Core elements of the marital bond are respect, trust, and intimacy. Respect lies in the spouses' acceptance of each other's weaknesses and vulnerabilities, as well as of their strengths and stellar characteristics. Trust is based on the belief that your spouse has your best interest in mind. Even when angry or disappointed, you trust that neither of you would purposely do something to hurt the other. Sexual intimacy is not the prime factor in marriage, but is a positive, integral part. The functions of sexuality are to share pleasure, to reinforce and strengthen intimacy, and to reduce tension in order to help couples cope with the stresses of job, children, house, and a shared life. When sex is problematic, it undermines the relationship and robs it of emotional energy. When sex functions well in a marriage, it contributes 15 to 20 percent to marital vitality. When it becomes dysfunctional or nonexistent it can drain 50 to 70 percent of the energy out of a relationship and rob the couple of trust and intimacy.

Alice and Brent's marital bond had been badly strained by frustration, discouragement, and misunderstanding, but it was still intact. As long as the marital bond is viable, sexual problems can be successfully dealt with. However, if the marital bond has been severed, it is hard to resurrect sex. Sex cannot save a non-viable relationship.

In therapy, the first focus was for Alice and Brent to view their sexual dysfunction as a couple problem. This allowed them to assume mutual responsibility and stop the blaming cycle. It also helped to establish a couple sexual style that was functional and satisfying for both Alice and Brent. Whether a new or revitalized relationship, you need to nurture comfort, attraction, and trust.

Alice and Brent found sex therapy very helpful. They were committed to revitalizing their intimate bond and willing to communicate and engage in sexual exercises to reach that goal. Progress was neither easy nor straightforward. Both positive experiences and learning from mistakes were necessary for them to rebuild and strengthen their couple sexual style. Alice and Brent realized sexual desire is not automatic. They needed to build bridges to desire, anticipate sexual encounters, stay away from behavior that poisoned desire, and set aside time to be a sexual couple rather than dream of the perfect spontaneous sex portrayed in movies. They were committed to nurturing desire and sexuality in their marriage.

Developing and Maintaining Sexual Intimacy

Becoming a sexual couple is a process that takes time and energy. A sexual relationship needs continual nurturing. It cannot rest on its laurels or be taken for granted. Comfort, attraction, and trust must be reinforced if desire and sexual satisfaction are to be maintained.

In traditional marital therapy, the sexual dysfunction is seen as a symptom of a relationship problem. If an underlying emotional problem in a relationship was successfully dealt with, so the reasoning went, the sexual dysfunction would spontaneously be cured. In fact, many couples have a trusting, respectful, caring relationship, but experience sexual problems due to lack of information, performance anxiety, poor sexual skills, poor sexual communication, or a history of unsuccessful experiences, guilt, and blaming. The more specific the sexual dysfunction, the greater the need to focus directly on sexual comfort and skills. The best examples are early ejaculation or ejaculatory inhibition in males and nonorgasmic response, arousal dysfunction, vaginismus, and sexual aversion in females.

Relationship problems can interfere with sexual functioning. Common problems include poor communication, lack of respect, anger over past events, frustration over relationship roles, power struggles, disappointments and resentments, disagreements about finances, child rearing conflicts, being turned off by the partner's behavior concerning drinking, eating, or cleanliness. Sometimes a problem revolves around a specific practical issue such as disparate times to go to sleep, not having a lock on the bedroom door, or conflict about contraceptive use. When couples become aware of complexly interwoven individual, relationship, and sexual problems, it is advisable to seek therapy.

Do not feel pressure to "keep up with the Joneses" sexually. Each couple develops their unique sexual style. It is crucial to put time and psychological energy into nurturing your intimate relationship. Key elements in reviving sexual desire are positive anticipation, building bridges to sexual desire, and the conviction that sexuality should be a pleasurable, satisfying part of your life and intimate relationship.

First Set of Exercises: Comfort

A first step in becoming a sexual couple is developing a comfortable, nondemand approach to sensuality. How can you enhance sexual comfort? Begin by setting aside at least two times, one in your bedroom and a second time in the family room, living room, or kitchen for this excercise. Although most of our exercises involve comfort with nudity, this exercise begins with clothes on.

Sensuality involves being receptive to and enjoying nondemand, non-genital touching. Sensuality means touching for its own sake, not as a goal toward arousal, intercourse, or orgasm. Being open to the joys of slow, tender, caring, rhythmic touching is the basis of sexual response and essential for maintaining a vital sexual relationship.

This exercise takes place in your bedroom with clothes on, with a focus on non-verbal communciation, and with the woman as initiator. Traditionally, women have not had permission to initiate sensual or sexual activities. She can initiate this excercise in the morning, in the late afternoon on a rainy weekend, or early in the evening (we suggest not doing it right before bed when you are tired and do not have the energy or concentration to explore). Begin by taking a bath or shower and playfully washing each other. Towel-dry your partner in a slow, caring fashion, and proceed to the bedroom. Put on clothing you feel comfortable with; it could be pajamas, a robe, or an informal outfit.

How personalized is your bedroom? Does it have personal mementos? Is it decorated the way you like? Is there sufficient light? Is it a comfortable room to be in? Orchestrate the milieu to increase sensuality. You could burn a fragrant candle. You could put music on the radio or stereo to romanticize the atmosphere. Be sure you are not too warm or cold.

Touch for yourself; do not try to second-guess your partner. Give yourself permission to experiment with a variety of ways of touching, holding, and caressing. Use your fingertips, palms, both hands, or only one. Do not limit yourself. Use your legs; rub your body against him; let your lips or tongue explore his body. He can take off as much or as little clothing as you prefer. Some couples find they are more comfortable if initially the man keeps his eyes closed; others enjoy keeping eye contact throughout. Try it both ways—which is more sensual? Explore and enjoy his body from the hairs on his head to the soles of his feet. Be aware of at least two areas you enjoy touching. Do not be surprised if there are body parts you do not like; this is not Tom

Cruise made up to look perfect on a movie screen, but your live partner with a scar on his kneecap, a roll of flab on his buttock, more hair than you like on his back.

Switch roles and let him explore your body to redevelop sensuality and comfort.

The bedroom is one thing; being comfortable in the kitchen, living room, or family room can be quite another. Do this part of the exercise in the next day or two. Since this exercise is done in the nude, ensure that you will have privacy and will not be interrupted by neighbors or children. An intimate relationship erodes because of lack of couple time. Couples discuss and problem-solve about practical, external problems, but have little time for personal, intimate feelings and communication.

Make this your special time. Would you rather talk in the kitchen, living room, or family room? Do you want a cup of tea or glass of wine? Would music in the background enhance or distract from communication? Sit comfortably, facing each other. Nonverbal components of communication, especially eye contact, body posture, facial response, and touch, carry a message as important as words. Is talking enhanced by holding hands, having your arm around your partner's shoulder, playfully touching your partner's hands or caressing your partner's face and neck?

How do you talk as a sexual couple? Is it comfortable to use proper words or employ slang; or do you have your private sexual language? Can you share emotional feelings and intimacy as easily as you make requests? Can you discuss what pleasuring and intercourse techniques increase sexual response? To be an intimate couple, you need to be able to discuss both emotional and sexual feelings.

Share your fondest memory of being sexual. Take the risk of being vulnerable and discuss how you felt during and after the experience.

The only time most couples are nude is in the bedroom while they are having sex. Being nude and touching and talking comfortably in the living room, den, or kitchen can be a liberating experience. Enjoy the freedom and openness of nude nondemand pleasuring and talking while nude outside the bedroom.

Is it helpful to touch while clothed in the bedroom? How do you feel about touching while nude outside the bedroom? Touching both inside and outside the bedroom is an excellent way to nurture sexual desire. Conclude the exercise by making requests that would make your sexual relationship, especially initiating sexual activity, comfortable and inviting.

Second Set of Exercises:
Couple Sexual Attraction

Sexual attraction is not a static property. It is not some "magic" quality that either you have or you don't. Sexual attraction is a dynamic process between two people that waxes and wanes. Attraction is affected by myriad factors. Physical attractiveness is but one factor; it is certainly not the only one or even the most important one. Turn-ons vary with each couple, contrary to the media myth that there is a perfect, youthful body type that turns everyone on. You can increase sexual attraction to each other and for each other.

Start this exercise clothed in a comfortable, private setting conducive to communication. Set aside at least forty-five minutes which could extend to a couple of hours if you wish. Present yourself in a manner that you feel is attractive; choose an outfit you particularly like, shave, fix your hair, brush your teeth, dab on your favorite perfume or after-shave—do the kinds of things people do for a date, but not in a relationship they unfortunately take for granted.

Discussing attraction can be awkward, so we suggest a semi-structured communication exercise. Let the woman begin. Tell your partner at least five things you find attractive about him, being as clear and specific as possible. You might find his slightly balding head attractive, his new glasses, the way he jogs, his arms and hands, how he looks in a suit and tie, his laugh, the tenderness he displays when putting the children to bed, how he handles a household emergency, the look in his eyes before initiating sex, how responsible he is about paying bills, the sounds he makes when he has an orgasm, his new-found skill at cooking casseroles, the muscles of his legs, how caring he was when his aunt died, how enraptured he is with classical music yet can still enjoy country, the way he stimulates you to arousal, how generous he can be with his time when someone needs help, his penis when he is aroused, how he puts up a tent when you go camping. Be honest in disclosing what you find attractive, physically, sexually, and psychologically. Be sure he is listening and acknowledging his positive qualities, not shrugging them off or minimizing them.

Now pick one, two, or at the most three things you want him to change which would increase his attractiveness. Do not just state the problem. Make a specific request for change. Say: "I'd like you to cut your hair one-and-a-half inches shorter and comb it at night," rather than: "I don't like your hair; do something about it." Say: "When you initiate, kiss me and stroke my arms before you touch my breasts," not: "You come on too strong." Say: "Talk and play with each child individually," rather than: "I get angry because you never pay attention to the kids."

Switch roles and have the man share what he finds attractive in his partner. He may like the way she wakes him up with a kiss, that other people view her as super-organized, how she purrs when her back is scratched, that she can fix broken items, the shape of her breasts, what a good athlete she is, how wet she becomes when she gets aroused, how she sings to the children before bedtime, how seductive she looks in a see-through nightgown, how she cheers him up after a bad day, how her nipple gets erect after he licks it, the way she pads around the house in bare feet, how attractive she looks when dressed for a night out, the care she takes planning family picnics, the effort she makes in picking clothes for the children, how she moves when she is sexually turned on, how assertive she is with neighbors. What is special about your partner that you value and find attractive?

In addressing the one to three changes, feel free to make them either sexual or nonsexual. What will increase your partner's attractiveness for you? Remember, it is a request, not a demand. Say: "I want you to sit with me once a month and plan big purchases," not: "You don't care anything about money except spending it." Say: "I want you to try orally stimulating me when I'm standing," not: "Stop being so hung up about oral sex!" Say: "I wish you would initiate sex by stroking my chest when you wake up on a weekend morning," rather than: "You never initiate."

After discussing the process of maintaining and enhancing attraction you can end the exercise or engage in touching which could lead to a sexual encounter.

Third Set of Exercises: Trust and Intimacy

One major value of an intimate relationship is the ability to trust that your partner is on your side, has your best interest in mind and would not do anything intentionally to hurt you. Trust is a central ingredient in an intimate relationship. Communicate how you feel about the level of trust, both in the past and at present. If it is not as high as you want, what can you do to increase it? What are the "trust vulnerabilities" the partner needs to be aware of? What can each of you do to increase trust? Trust is not something that occurs automatically; it takes time to allow feelings of trust and intimacy to develop and be expressed both verbally and physically.

Couples can establish a "trust" or "safe" sexual position where they feel cared about and secure. This involves being nude in the privacy of your bedroom. Can you personalize your bedroom—have a special light that gives a warm glow, a favorite erotic book or love poem by the bedstand, thick curtains so there is privacy, a full-length mirror to increase visual stimuli? Do you enjoy lying and talking in your bedroom? Caress your partner's face and recall a time when you felt vulnerable and your partner was there for you.

You have experimented with nondemand positions to increase receptivity, sensuality, and responsiveness. Develop a "safe" or "trust" position that facilitates feelings of intimacy and trust. You might lie side by side holding each other, your bodies touching from the tips of your toes to your forehead. Try a position where the male partner is sitting up with his back supported and the woman is lying with her head on his lap while he strokes her hair as they talk. Another trust position is lying next to each other, holding hands and being silent. Some couples use a "spoon" position where the woman lies with her chest against her partner's back, puts her arms around him, and breathes in unison with his rhythm. In another position, the man lies on his back and the woman nestles her head against his shoulder; their faces are close so they can maintain good eye contact. A trust position some couples value is sitting facing each other, keeping eye contact, putting one hand on the partner's heart. What adds to your sense of trust—body contact, eye contact, being comfortable, feeling secure, being enveloped, talking, silence? Find at least one position where you feel intimate and trusting.

In subsequent sexual experiences, when you become anxious, depressed, frustrated, or angry, utilize this trust position as a "port in the storm." Rather than ending a sexual exercise on an anxious or frustrated note, switch to your trust position as a way of anchoring yourself. You can choose whether to continue the exercise or end the experience from your trust position. This helps you remain connected and realize you can depend on each other. You trust you are an intimate team.

Fourth Set of Exercises: Couple Sexual Scenario

When a relationship is new, there is strong anticipation of being sexual, even if the quality of sex is not particularly good. Sex serves as an affirmation of your desirability and desire to be a couple. Romantic love and passionate sex energize a relationship and make it "magical." There is the thrill of sexual exploration as well as energy that goes into making the relationship an exciting, loving experience.

After the initial romantic love/passionate sex has dissipated, it takes most couples six months to develop a sexual style that is functional, intimate, and satisfying. Part of the process is the development of couple sexual scenarios, the focus of this exercise. As a reminder, you are not a machine so it is normal in the best of couples to occasionally have mediocre or negative sexual experiences. A sign of a healthy couple is their ability to accept and not overreact to negative experiences.

What do you value most in a sexual experience? Each individual develops her/his sexual scenario. Let the woman introduce her scenario first. At another time the man can develop his.

When is your best time to be sexual? Waking up? After the morning paper? At noon? Before or after a nap? Before dinner (sex as an appetizer) or after dinner (sex as dessert)? In the evening? Most couples have sex late at night, but interestingly, few people say this is their favorite time. How do you set your preferred sensual and sexual mood? Do you listen to music, go for a walk, talk, light candles and drink wine, take a bath, have fifteen minutes of time alone and then come together, meet your partner at the door and seduce him into the bedroom? As a prelude to being sexual some couples enjoy doing together things like shopping, working in the garden, going for a run, sharing feelings. Many couples start touching and playing in the living room or den and do not move on to the bedroom until both are turned on. Others prefer to start in the privacy of their bedroom. What is your favorite way to begin a sexual scenario? Remember, there is no right or wrong—it is your preference.

Once the scenario is under way, what is your favorite script? Do you like to take turns or would you prefer mutual stimulation? Do you verbally express sexual feelings or would you rather let your fingers do the talking? Do you prefer a slow build-up or would you rather begin intercourse as soon as you are aroused? Do you like multiple stimulation or one erotic focus at a time? Do you make use of all your senses—touch, taste, smell, hearing, sight—or does one element (observing the sex flush, hearing soft moans, smelling an erotic perfume, feeling sexual movement) turn you on? Develop the scenario the way you want. Your partner is open to your guidance.

How would you like to end the scenario? Afterplay is the most neglected element of the sexual experience. Your needs and desires are important here, too. Do you like to lie and hold your partner, sleep in each other's arms, engage in playful tickling, have a warm kiss, take a walk, read poetry, nap and start again, talk and come down together?

When it is the man's turn to create a sexual scenario, he can feel free to design his own, which could be similar to or totally different from hers. Many men fall into the trap of trying to outdo their partner. Sex is neither a competition nor a performance. Be yourself; develop an initiation, script, and afterplay which is erotic and special.

Guidelines for Revitalizing and Maintaining
Sexual Desire

These guidelines are used to enhance sexual desire and prevent relapse.

1. Essential keys to sexual desire are positive anticipation and feeling that you deserve sexual pleasure.
2. The process of change involves a one–two combination of assuming personal responsibility and being an intimate team. Each person is responsible for his or her desire with the couple functioning as an intimate team to nurture and enhance desire. Revitalizing sexual desire is a couple task. Guilt, blame, and pressure subvert the change process.
3. Inhibited desire is the most common sexual dysfunction, affecting two in five couples. Sexual avoidance drains intimacy and vitality from the marital bond.
4. One in five married couples has a non-sexual relationship (being sexual less than ten times a year). One in three unmarried couples who have been together longer than two years has a non-sexual relationship.
5. The average frequency of sexual intercourse is between four times a week to once every two weeks. For couples in their twenties, the average sexual frequency is two to three times a week; for couples in their fifties, once a week.
6. The initial romantic love/passionate sex kind of desire lasts less than two years and usually less than six months. Desire is facilitated by an emotionally intimate, interactive relationship.
7. Contrary to the myth that "horniness" occurs after not being sexual for weeks, desire is facilitated by a regular rhythm of sexual activity. When sex occurs less than twice a month, couples become self-conscious and fall into a cycle of anticipatory anxiety, tense and unsatisfying sex, and avoidance.
8. A key strategy is to develop "her," "his," and "our" bridges to sexual desire. This involves ways of thinking, talking, anticipating, and feeling that invite sexual encounters.

9. The essence of sexuality is giving and receiving pleasure-oriented touching. The prescription for maintaining desire is to integrate intimacy, pleasuring, and eroticism.

10. Touching occurs both inside and outside the bedroom, and is valued for itself. Both the man and woman can be comfortable initiating. Touching should not always lead to intercourse. Both partners can feel free to say "no" and to suggest an alternative way to connect and share pleasure.

11. Couples who maintain a vital sexual relationship can use as a metaphor for touching "five gears." First gear is clothes-on, affectionate touch (holding hands, kissing, hugging). Second gear is non-genital, sensual touch, which can be done clothed, semi-clothed, or nude (body massage, cuddling on the couch, showering together, touching while going to sleep or on awakening). Third gear is playful touch, which intermixes genital and non-genital touching, clothed or unclothed, and may take place in bed, while dancing, in the shower, or on the couch. Fourth gear is erotic touch (manual, oral, or rubbing) and may lead to arousal and orgasm for one or both partners. Fifth gear integrates pleasurable with erotic touch and flows into intercourse.

12. Personal turn-ons facilitate sexual anticipation and desire. These include the use of fantasy and erotic scenarios, as well as sex associated with special celebrations or anniversaries, sex with the goal of conception, sex when feeling caring and close, or even sex to soothe a personal disappointment.

13. External turn-ons (R- or X-rated videos, music, candles, sexy clothing, visual feedback from mirrors, locations other than the bedroom, a weekend away without the kids) can elicit sexual desire.

14. Males and females with hormonal deficits may use testosterone injections, patches, or creams to enhance sexual desire, but only under medical supervision. Medical problems and side-effects of other medications can interfere with sexual desire and function.

15. Sexuality has a number of positive functions—as a shared pleasure, as a means to reinforcing and deepening intimacy, and as a tension reducer to deal with the stresses of life and marriage.

16. "Intimate coercion" is not acceptable. Sexuality is neither a reward nor a punishment. Healthy sexuality is voluntary, mutual, and pleasure-oriented.

17. Realistic expectations are crucial for maintaining a healthy sexual relationship. It is self-defeating to demand equal desire, arousal, orgasm and satisfaction each time. A positive, realistic expectation is that 40 to 50 percent of experiences are very good for both people; 20 to 25 percent are very good for one partner (usually the man) and fine for the other; 20 to 25 percent are acceptable but not remarkable. 5 to 15 percent of sexual experiences are mediocre or failures. Couples who accept this without guilt or blaming and try again when they are receptive and responsive will have a vital, resilient sexual relationship. Satisfied couples use the guideline of "good-enough" sex.

18. If the couple has gone two weeks without any sexual contact, the partner with higher desire should take the initiative to set up a planned or spontaneous sexual date. If that does not occur, the other partner should initiate a sensual or play date during the following week. If that does not occur and they have gone a month without sexual contact, they should schedule a "booster" therapy session.

19. Healthy sexual desire plays a positive, integral role in an intimate relationship, its main function being to energize the bond and generate special feelings. Paradoxically, bad or non-existent sex plays a more powerful negative role in a relationship than the positive role of good sex.

Closing Thoughts

Developing a couple sexual style and building bridges to sexual desire are crucial. Even more important, and more difficult, is maintaining a healthy sexual desire and satisfying sexual relationship. Emotional and sexual intimacy needs continual nurturing. The most important guideline is to set aside "couple time" to be together and share feelings rather than just dealing with the practical concerns of jobs, house, children, and money. If sexuality is to remain vital and satisfying, it requires communication, spontaneity, experimentation, and a sense of playfulness. Make your intimate relationship a priority.

Sex is not the most important component in a couple relationship, but it is integral and special. Sexuality functions as a shared pleasure, a means to build and reinforce intimacy, and a tension-reducer to help deal with the hassles of everyday living. A vital sexual life energizes and makes a special marital bond. If sex is allowed to stagnate, it devitalizes the relationship. You have invested a good deal in becoming a sexual couple; continue to devote the time and energy to maintain sexual desire and intimacy.

15

Increasing Female Arousal

Until the last generation, it was assumed that men were infinitely more sexually desirous and responsive than women. Sex was the woman's duty, not her pleasure. At best, according to the traditional view, sex was tolerated because it allowed affection and intimacy. The woman was not expected to anticipate sexual intercourse, or to enjoy it. After all, sex was painful and degrading. And the idea that women could enjoy sex more than men was heretical.

In truth, empirical research has found many more similarities than differences in female and male sexual response. Females and males have similar capacities for desire, pleasure, arousal, orgasm and satisfaction. Actually, women have the opportunity to be more sexually expressive because they have the potential to have several orgasms—to be multi-orgasmic.

Women now can give themselves permission to enjoy healthy, normal sexuality. Sexuality is as worthwhile for them as for men. A couple that is comfortable with emotional intimacy, pleasuring, and eroticism will find that sexuality reinforces their intimate relationship. Traditional female sexual socialization emphasized intimacy and non-demand pleasuring, but not eroticism. Valuing eroticism is an integral component of vital female sexuality.

New Myths Replace Old Myths

In helping the woman understand, accept, and enjoy her sexuality, the goal is *not* to foster competition between partners. "The War Between the Sexes" has done great damage to women and men. Both the woman and man need to be sexually aware so that they can share and enhance their communication and sexual expression. Massive misunderstandings regarding female sexuality have proved to be a major inhibiting factor in the development of a couple's intimate relationship. Unfortunately, findings about female sexuality, especially orgasm, have not been well presented by the media. Sensationalistic articles and case reports have resulted in new myths, such as the belief the woman *must* have an orgasm each time, the tenet that orgasm is the *only* measure of satisfaction, the myth of the primacy of the "G" spot, or the belief that being multi-orgasmic is superior to having a single orgasm.

The crucial fact is that female sexual response is more complex and variable than male response. It is not better or worse, more sexual or less sexual, but is more flexible and variable.

Variations in Arousal

Typically, the male has one orgasm during intercourse. Although there is considerable variability in psychological feelings of enjoyment and satisfaction, male orgasm is a stereotyped response. Not so the female sexual response. The woman may have no orgasm, one, or many. Orgasm might occur during pleasuring/foreplay, intercourse, or afterplay. There can also be considerable variation in the woman's feelings of satisfaction. For example, there are times a woman might enjoy sex a great deal even though she is non-orgasmic. Orgasm in and of itself is not a good measure of sexual satisfaction. This is not to say that orgasm is less important; it is a positive, integral component of female sexuality. However, it should not become a performance demand, nor should it be used as a test of femininity.

"Sophisticated" males feel they have failed as lovers if their partner is not orgasmic each time. This is as harmful a sexual myth as the old myth that females were not supposed to enjoy sex. Orgasm is the natural culmination of sexual involvement and arousal; it cannot be willed or demanded. A woman is a sexual person, not a perfectly predictable sexual machine. The more the woman (and her partner) work to achieve orgasm, the less likely it is to occur. Female orgasmic dysfunction is caused by demands and pressure (from herself or partner) in the same manner that a male's erectile dysfunction is often caused by performance anxiety.

Learning to be aroused and orgasmic is a gradually developed skill as the woman and couple understand, accept, and enhance her sexuality and their sexual functioning. Arousal and orgasm are not mysterious processes that must be conquered to prove a woman is sexual. Through self-exploration exercises and non-genital and genital pleasuring experiences, you have established a base of understanding and acceptance. Exercises in this chapter build on and extend that base. The focus is on pleasure, eroticism, and arousal. The next chapter will focus specifically on orgasm.

Very few females (less than 5 percent) learn orgasmic response during intercourse. The great majority have their first orgasm through masturbation, by manual stimulation, with the use of a vibrator, through cunnilingus or during afterplay. Physiologically, an orgasm is the same whether achieved through masturbation, vibrator stimulation, cunnilingus, manual stimulation, rubbing stimulation or intercourse. Scientifically, the distinction between "vaginal" and "clitoral" orgasms is untrue. Orgasm is a response to indirect clitoral stimulation and is experienced as muscle contractions in the vulva. This is true whether the penis is in the vagina or stimulation is through hands, tongue, rubbing, or vibrator. There are differences in psychological satisfaction, depending on expectations, values, preferences, and partner response.

Jan and Mel

Jan was forty-three, divorced three years ago, and married to Mel for five months. Jan was orgasmic on self-stimulation and was often orgasmic during partner sex. As soon as intercourse ended, Mel asked whether Jan had an orgasm—which was a major turn-off for her. If she said yes, whether true or not, Mel felt he had fulfilled his masculine role. Jan was less worried about orgasm (although she certainly enjoyed and valued orgasm), and more concerned about her difficulty feeling responsive and becoming aroused.

Jan had read a good deal about female sexuality and wanted to communicate her feelings and concerns to Mel before their sexual relationship became a major problem. She felt comfortable with and attracted to Mel. Jan was committed to making this a satisfying, stable marriage. The question was whether she could trust him to be sexually cooperative and giving. Some men see the woman's sexual difficulty as a personal challenge, which puts a tremendous performance demand on her (and on him). If she does not perform according to his expectations, he will berate her for being "frigid." When a sexual difficulty is not resolved, the man in most cases blames the woman and thus adds to her self-blame and the feeling that she is "defective."

Mel listened in an understanding, respectful manner and said he wanted to be there for her and share sexual pleasure. Mel was not responsible for "turning her on," but was open to her guidance and requests. Jan needed to be her own person and take responsibility for her arousal, to develop her "sexual voice." She wanted to be free to express herself (make requests, utter sounds, move her body) without fear of being judged by Mel. Typically it takes six months for a couple to develop a sexual style which is comfortable and satisfying. For Mel and Jan, it took ten months, but was well worth the time and energy invested.

Both partners in an intimate relationship need to increase awareness of the woman's sexual receptivity and responsivity pattern. The emphasis should not be on orgasm, but on increasing pleasure, eroticism and arousal. If the woman is orgasmic, that is fine; orgasm is the natural culmination of increased sexual involvement, pleasure, eroticism and arousal.

Increasing eroticism and arousal is a mutual experience—not one for the woman to do alone or for the man to do for her.

First Set of Exercises: Trust

This exercise focuses on increasing sexual trust. The dating patterns in our culture teach the female not to trust the male, but to be guarded and defensive in her sexual expression. She learns not to show arousal because of fear that he would take advantage of her. Many, in fact most, women have felt disappointed or hurt in sexual relationships. Such experience further builds the wall of vigilance and distrust. Whether the negative experience was being harassed, humiliated, or raped, our culture has long condoned sexual mistreatment and abuse of women. Such cultural attitudes and negative feelings inhibit sexual expression for the woman even though she is now in an intimate relationship. So, at the onset of this exercise, talk about how your trust has grown as a result of the nondemand sensual and genital pleasuring exercises. Note especially the importance of giving and utilizing feedback, verbal and non-verbal.

Start by bathing together. The male can be particularly indulgent of the woman's feelings, washing her gently and tenderly. Take a big, fluffy towel and pat her dry. To accentuate feelings of trust, she can close her eyes and let him lead her to the bedroom, with the feeling that she is safe and cared for.

Assume the pleasuring position called the "vulnerability" or "trust" position. The man positions himself comfortably against a wall, bedboard, or cushions, with his legs spread. The woman positions her back against his chest and her legs within his. She can place her head on his shoulder. His hands have easy access to her neck, breasts, stomach, vulva, and thighs.

Both partners should keep their eyes closed so they can focus on warm, intimate, trusting feelings. The man's touch should be slow, tender, caring, and rhythmic. As her comfort increases, he can gently open her legs and put them over his. There is almost total body contact. This can facilitate emotional and sexual intimacy.

With her legs spread, the woman's vulva is open and exposed. A woman is taught not to sit that way, yet being open and receptive is totally healthy in an intimate relationship. She should focus on feeling cared for and trusting, so different from feeling vulnerable and

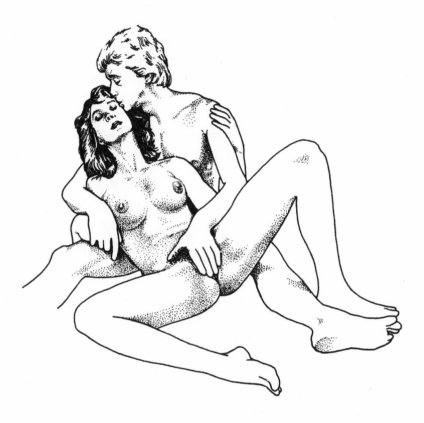

The "trust" position for sexual stimulation of the female.

inhibited. She can allow herself to feel responsive and experience pleasure and arousal.

Pleasuring intermixes non-genital and genital touching, with the rhythm of touching in unison with the woman's pace and arousal. Utilize pleasurable stimulation in the context of a nondemanding, trusting, and caring connection. As the woman becomes responsive and aroused, continue the rhythm of stimulation. A mistake males often make is to increase the speed or depth of stimulation to try to bring her to orgasm. Instead, she loses her rhythm and arousal, she no longer feels into an erotic flow. She feels frustrated and demanded upon, while the male feels he has failed as a lover or blames her for being non-responsive. Key to female eroticism, arousal and orgasm is continued stimulation given in a consistent rhythm. The male follows the woman's movements and rhythm. She is the expert on her body, arousal, and sexual response.

If the woman does not become aroused, her partner should accept this. She may simply enjoy the sensuous, trusting, and caring feelings. The focus, after all, is to build feelings of trust and comfort without a sexual demand.

End this exercise by breathing together. The man is comfortably on his side, the woman's head against his upper back and her breasts touching his back. She can follow the rhythm of his breathing. As you breathe together, be aware of intimate, trusting feelings. Verbally share these feelings and allow yourselves to drift off to sleep. The core ingredients for female sexual response—sense of trust, receptivity and responsiveness without demand or inhibitions—are now on solid footing. Intimacy, trust, and pleasuring are not sufficient for arousal and orgasm, but are necessary.

Second Set of Exercises: Vulva Exploration

The woman can share, as specifically as possible, her conditions for being receptive and responsive to sexual stimulation. Her taking responsibility for her "sexual voice" is essential to increasing arousal. She should verbalize her desire for sharing erotic and arousing sexual experiences. It is easy for a woman to be distracted and turn off sexually. She can tell her partner what to avoid so this does not happen inadvertently. If in the midst of a sexual interaction she does lose erotic flow and arousal, return to comfortable, pleasurable touching. Most women are able to regain receptivity and arousal, others find it difficult. At a later time, outside the bedroom, the couple can discuss how to deal with the waxing and waning of arousal in a cooperative, pleasurable manner rather than in an angry, resentful or accusatory mode.

Start with a bath or shower. Make it a relaxing, sharing experience. The male begins as pleasure-giver. The woman may keep her eyes open to facilitate communication or, if she wishes, close them to be in touch with her bodily sensations and feelings. Arrange yourselves in a position where the man leans against either the headboard or wall with his back supported by a pillow or cushion. She positions her body between his spread legs, lying on her back and facing him, with her legs bent and resting outside his thighs. He has easy access to her open vulva as well as her breasts. She can touch him if she desires, but her focus should be on accepting touch and building her pleasure and arousal.

The man begins by touching his partner non-genitally, in a slow, tender, rhythmic manner. Genital touching is gradually integrated with non-genital. The woman can guide him by putting her hand over his, modifying her movements, or making verbal requests to alter the rhythm of touching. By making clear requests, the woman takes responsibility for her pleasure. The man might use a light, teasing touch, moving from her neck to vulva, then around her abdomen and thighs in a flowing movement, and on to her breasts, using the type of breast stimulation he has learned is pleasing. Touching should cover her entire body and not be focused on her vulva.

Vulva stimulation can begin as light and teasing. As the woman becomes aroused and begins to lubricate, the man gently puts one or two fingers in the vagina. Spread the vaginal lubrication throughout the vulva, especially around the clitoral area. Continue non-genital and genital pleasuring. Neither partner demands or forces; both accentuate their sensual and erotic feelings.

The clitoris is the area of most nerve endings and erotic sensations. The only function of the clitoris is sexual pleasure. Exploration of the clitoral area can be confusing because the clitoris is small and during arousal is covered by the clitoral hood. The woman can take her partner's hand and guide him in touching and stroking her labia. She can take his finger and move it around her clitoral area in a gentle, exploratory manner. Most women prefer indirect stimulation around the clitoral shaft rather than direct clitoral stimulation, which can be too intense and even painful (the clitoris going under the clitoral hood is her body's way to facilitate pleasure and avoid pain).

Many women react negatively to vaginal insertion; it can be a turn-off if there is little arousal. It would be as if the woman rhythmically stroked the man's penis when it was flaccid. Rather than building arousal, it increases self-consciousness and irritation. Too often men initiate vaginal insertion and then forget about other pleasuring techniques. Most women find vaginal pleasuring to be stimulating when there is at least a moderate level of arousal and a focus at the same time on additional pleasuring, especially clitoral and breast stimulation.

With his index finger, the man can explore intravaginally to help the woman identify and discriminate areas of vaginal feeling and response. She closes her eyes so she can focus on vaginal sensations. While exploring the vagina with one hand, he continues sensuous non-genital touching with his other. If at any time either partner feels pressured or uncomfortable, return to non-genital pleasuring.

You can conceptualize the vagina as a clock with the section closest to the clitoris as twelve o'clock and the part closest to the anus as six o'clock. The man can insert his index finger within the vagina to approximately two finger joints. Contrary to the popular myth (the deeper the insertion, the greater the feeling), insertion of two finger joints—about one and one-half inches—reaches the section of the vagina adjacent to the pubococcygeal muscle, an area of intense vaginal sensation. Contrary to the myth about a magical "G" spot as the source of vaginal orgasm, the anterior wall of the vagina, when stimulated, increases arousal for many (but not all) women.

The man can gently but firmly move his index finger (or a second finger, if the woman so desires) around the vagina. This movement should be slow so she can identify sensations and feelings. She can give verbal and nonverbal feedback to guide him during intravaginal stimulation. Touching certain areas of the vagina can be uncomfortable or painful. This might be due to tears in the vaginal wall or due to vaginal dryness. Discomfort can be alleviated by using a lubricant and/or exercises to strengthen the pubococcygeal muscle. If the woman does experience chronic pain, she should consult her gynecologist. Vaginal pain can be caused by infection, physical abnormalities, or estrogen deprivation. Vaginismus is a sexual dysfunction that involves the spasming of the vaginal introitus (opening) so intromission is either impossible or painful. Pelvic or vaginal pain is a frequent sexual complaint that needs to be assessed by a gynecologist. It is most likely to be successfully treated by using sexual exercises under the guidance of a sex therapist.

Vaginal pain often reflects lack of arousal and lubrication or the man's being rough and demanding rather than open to the woman's feedback and requests. Use of a hypoallergenic lotion or estrogen cream can enhance lubrication. Gynecologists recommend K-Y jelly because it is sterile, but many women prefer abalone lotion, aloe vera lotion, or another pleasant smelling lotion from the drug store or a specialty store. Be sure the lotion is water-based and will not irritate or infect the vagina.

Stimulation of specific sections of the vagina can be sexually arousing. Some women find stimulation of two finger joints at four o'clock and eight o'clock particularly erotic. Others report greater vaginal feeling with pressure on the anterior wall. Some women report relatively little intravaginal feeling. There is no right or normal response. What counts are your sensations and feelings.

The woman can tell her partner to stop when she feels aware and comfortable with vulva, clitoral and intravaginal sensations and feelings. You might do this excercise once or try it on several occasions, using different positions to explore clitoral and vaginal responsiveness. Most women find they enjoy clitoral, labia, and mons stimulation more than vaginal stimulation. Experiment with different combinations of touch, rhythm, and pressure. What is your pattern of sexual receptivity and responsiveness? Feel free to discuss and experiment with erotic scenarios and techniques to increase vulva, clitoral and vaginal responsiveness.

Third Set of Exercises: Multiple Stimulation

This exercise includes use of a lotion to increase sensual feelings. Choose a lotion you enjoy the touch and smell of. Pleasuring can begin with the partners lying facing each other. Both can keep their eyes open.

Intermix non-genital and genital pleasuring and integrating what you have learned from previous exercises. It is particularly important for the woman to feel free in guiding her partner toward the manual and/or oral stimulation she finds most pleasurable and erotic. Continue stimulation until the woman feels excitement and arousal. Check to see if she wants to increase erotic stimulation. Checking out and feedback can be verbal (saying: "Do you feel into it?" or: "Is this arousing?") or nonverbal (touching her vulva, using your hand to close her eyes, using a signal you mutually agree on). If she responds in the negative, continue pleasuring, allowing it to be mutual, and then ending the experience in a sensual manner. Afterward, discuss what each of you can do to facilitate comfort, trust, sensuality, and eroticism.

If the woman's response is positive, the man can get on his knees and kneel over her from a side position. He can then help her move into a comfortable, receptive position, i.e., stretch her legs out, put a pillow under her head, place her arm by her side. He can orally stimulate (by kissing, licking, or taking small bites) from the top of her head to her mons. At the same time, he can manually stimulate from the mons to the bottoms of her feet. Stimulation can begin as light and teasing, then in a natural, rhythmic, and, most important, *slow* flow, become focused, directed, and erotic. He can orally stimulate her breasts by kissing, licking, or sucking while at the same time manually stimulating the labia and clitoral shaft. If she finds manual intravaginal

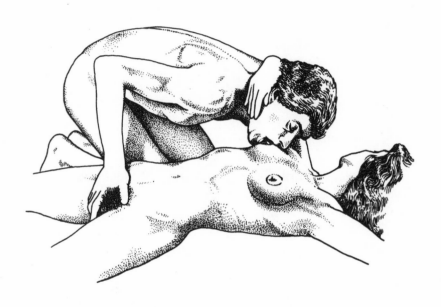

Multiple stimulation to heighten sexual responsiveness of the female.

stimulation arousing, that too can be added. Some women find the pressure of finger stimulation inside the vagina (especially the anterior wall) adds to arousal if they are already aroused—if not, it can be irritating and a turn-off. Stimulation should be consistent, in rhythm with the woman's movements and feelings. She should feel free to direct his touching and set the rhythm. Remember, it is *her* arousal and response pattern.

Contrary to the myth of male responsibility for sex, no one knows more about female eroticism and arousal than the woman. Neither partner should demand or force sexual response. Arousal and eroticism are the natural result of accepting, guiding, requesting, and building on sensual and sexual feelings. The woman should give herself permission to let go with abandon to eroticism and arousal. She can be "sexually selfish" and allow herself to be aroused, responsive, and expressive. She can and should enjoy eroticism.

Fourth Set of Exercises: Quiet Vagina

You might sit over a drink or cup of coffee and discuss the attitudinal and behavioral changes you have experienced thus far. What are your feelings about female sexuality and eroticism? Share feelings, perceptions, experiences, hopes, feelings, desires. Does the male feel comfortable with the woman's arousal or is he threatened by it? Is she trusting and accepting of erotic feelings or does she feel vulnerable or inhibited? Is orgasm a goal of overwhelming importance or is it a natural consequence of sexual responsiveness? Are receptivity, pleasure, eroticism, arousal, and orgasm a natural, flowing process or is it the big performance (The Big "O") for which you pressure yourself? Are you comfortable being active and responsible for your sexuality? Have you stopped trying to prove something to yourself or your partner?

Begin this exercise with mutual pleasuring, using non-genital and genital touching as well as manual and oral stimulation. Allow feelings of sexual responsivity and arousal to build. Develop a comfortable, pleasurable, erotic rhythm. Allow each partner's arousal to be a turn-on for the other. Sometimes the woman is the initiator and pleasure-giver, sometimes the male, but usually there is mutual stimulation. Utilize slow, tender, caring, rhythmic, flowing touching to increase feelings of openness and receptivity. It is exciting to be aware of and enjoy the responsivity of your partner; enjoy this variation on the give-to-get pleasuring guideline. See each other's arousal as a plus, not as a competition or pressure to keep up.

When both partners are feeling aroused, move to the female-on-top intercourse position. Avoid immediate intromission. Explore sensations and feelings; the woman might play with her partner's penis around her vulva. This is a good position for both verbal and nonverbal communication. It gives the woman a greater range of movement than other intercourse positions. It enables the man to stimulate her breasts as well as touch and caress her thighs while she takes his penis and rubs it around her labia, clitoral shaft, and vaginal opening. Be together as a couple; enjoy receiving and giving pleasure. Let the woman determine when to initiate intromission; she can wait until she is feeling highly aroused and desirous. Many women (and men) initiate intercourse too early in the arousal cycle.

Intromission is accomplished by sliding back on the penis at a forty-five degree angle. Allow her to guide intromission. Once intromission occurs, practice the "quiet vagina" exercise. The woman guides the penis to the most sensitive parts of her vagina and enjoys penile sensations with minimal movement. She can engage in slow, nondemand thrusting to maintain arousal. She should be aware of feelings in the vagina and throughout her body. She should think of his penis as something to play with.

The quiet vagina can also be enjoyed by the man, who can feel the wet warmth of the vagina and enjoy slow, nondemanding sensations. Continue the quiet vagina for five to ten minutes, longer if you wish. During this time, touch each other; be aware of a range of sensual and sexual feelings, especially feelings of being cared for and sharing sexuality.

During this time, or in subsequent experiences, you can proceed from the quiet vagina to active thrusting. However, resist reverting back to the old intercourse pattern. Slowly increase the amount of

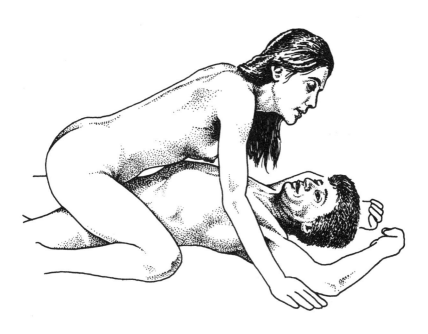

The "quiet vagina" exercise position to enhance sexual
expressiveness of the female.

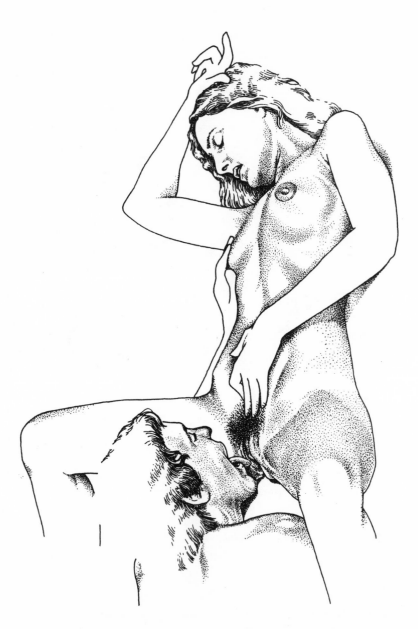

Oral stimulation of the female: an "orgasm trigger."

movement. Allow her to initiate and guide the rhythm and type of coital thrusting.

In subsequent exercises, experiment with different movements and positions and enjoy the variety of sensations. You can experiment with in-and-out thrusting, circular thrusting or up-and-down thrusting. You can vary the speed and rhythm of movement. You can try the side-by-side, man-on-top, and rear-entry intercourse positions. She might contract her pubococcygeal muscle while the penis is inside her. She can be fully accepting of the feelings of his penis in her vagina.

During intercourse he can stimulate her clitoral area manually while his penis is in her. Many couples find simultaneous clitoral and vaginal stimulation adds to eroticism and sexual responsiveness. Experiment with several variations—he can use his hand, she can use her hand, or you can utilize vibrator stimulation.

Afterward, discuss the quiet vagina experience. The woman can share what she particularly enjoyed—her reaction to his penis, initiating intercourse, guiding intromission, the slower thrusting, multiple stimulation during intercourse, combining vaginal and clitoral stimulation. The man can share his feelings—how it felt to be passive during intercourse, how her vagina felt to his penis, how to incorporate multiple stimulation during intercourse, variations of woman-on-top and other intercourse positions he would like to experiment with. He can reassure his partner that her being sexually active and assertive is not a sexual threat or turn-off. Be aware how you as a couple can integrate multiple stimulation, before and during intercourse.

Guidelines for Female Arousal and Orgasm

These guidelines are used to facilitate female sexual functioning and prevent release.

1. A woman is responsible for her desire, arousal and orgasm. Developing your "sexual voice" is a positive challenge. It is not the man's responsibility to "give you" an orgasm.

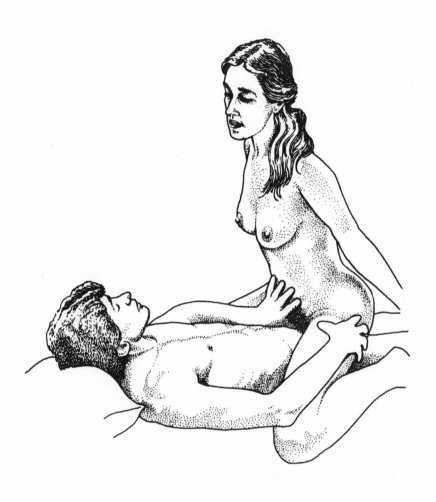

Clitoral stimulation during female-superior intercourse.

2. Together the couple develop an intimate, interactive sexual style that promotes desire, arousal, orgasm, and satisfaction for both partners.

3. Receptivity and responsivity to giving and receiving pleasurable and erotic touch is essential to arousal and orgasm.

4. Arousal involves both subjective components (feeling responsive and turned on) and objective components (vaginal lubrication and physical receptivity to intercourse).

5. Eroticism and high arousal includes intercourse, but is not limited to intercourse.

6. "Foreplay" where the man stimulates the woman to get her ready for intercourse increases self-consciousness and performance anxiety. The experience of "pleasuring" which emphasizes mutuality and sharing facilitates involvement and arousal.

7. The prescription for satisfying sexuality is integrating intimacy, pleasuring, and eroticism. Traditionally, female sexual socialization underplayed eroticism. Erotic scenarios and techniques are integral to female sexuality.

8. As you develop your "sexual voice," increase awareness of the erotic scenarios and techniques that enhance arousal. Use that awareness to make requests and guide your partner, verbally and non-verbally.

9. State your preferences—single vs. multiple stimulation, taking turns vs. mutual stimulation; when and how to proceed from sensual to erotic stimulation; your emotional and practical conditions for a vital sexual relationship. Feel free to request erotic techniques (vibrator stimulation, his or her fingers for clitoral stimulation during intercourse, cunnilingus to orgasm).

10. You can initiate the transition from pleasuring to intercourse and guide intromission.

11. Women who prefer multiple stimulation during pleasuring/ eroticism usually prefer multiple stimulation during intercourse. You can utilize additional clitoral stimulation with your hand or his, request breast or anal stimulation, fantasize, kiss, and/or switch intercourse positions.

12. Many women are interested in using medication, especially Viagra and/or testosterone, to enhance sexual response. Medication can be a valuable additional resource, but is not a "magic answer."

13. Many women use some form of estrogen and/or a water based lubricant to enhance lubrication and facilitate intercourse.

14. Only one in four women follow the traditional male pattern of one orgasm during intercourse. Female sexual response is flexible and variable. A woman may be non-orgasmic, singly orgasmic, or multi-orgasmic. Orgasm can occur during pleasuring, intercourse, or afterplay.

15. Sexuality is about experiencing and sharing pleasure. Sex is not a performance in order to achieve a "G" spot orgasm, multiple orgasms, "vaginal" orgasm, extended orgasm, or whatever is the new fad. Each woman develops her pattern of desire, arousal, and orgasm.

16. Orgasm is a three to ten second experience. Orgasm is a natural result of giving yourself permission to enjoy eroticism, arousal, and letting go so that arousal flows to orgasm.

17. The distinction between a "clitoral" and "vaginal" orgasm is not scientifically valid. Whether orgasm occurs with manual or oral stimulation, by rubbing, intercourse, or vibrator stimulation, the physiological response is the same. Subjective feelings of satisfaction vary depending on preferences, experiences, and values.

18. Desire and emotional satisfaction are more important than orgasm.

19. It is unrealistic to expect arousal and orgasm during each sexual experience. You are not a sexual machine. Female sexuality is more variable and complex than male sexuality.

20. Remember, sexuality is not about proving anything to your partner, yourself, or anyone else. It is about sharing and enjoying intimacy, pleasure, and eroticism.

Closing Thoughts

As a woman and a couple you can be comfortable and accepting of vital integrated female sexuality. Awareness, pleasure, and arousal continue to grow as you integrate sensual, playful, erotic and intercourse experiences. It is important that both people understand and accept the complexity of female sexual response. Intimacy and mutual satisfaction are much better criteria of sexual satisfaction than just orgasm.

16

Becoming Orgasmic

emale orgasm, "The Big O." There has been more talk and articles written about orgasm than any other area of sexual functioning. Are you less of a woman if you do not have an orgasm each time you have sex? Are multiple orgasms better than single orgasms? Is simultaneous orgasm the ideal? Are there differences between vaginal and clitoral orgasms? Is the "G" spot orgasm the best? Is it the man's responsibility to give the woman an orgasm? Old myths are replaced by new myths.

Here are some scientifically and clinically valid facts and guidelines. Orgasm is integral to the comfort/pleasure/arousal cycle, not something separate from it. Orgasm is the natural culmination of involved, effective sexual stimulation. Orgasm is a psychophysiological response and a positive, integral part of female sexuality. The physical orgasmic response is a series of genital muscle contractions which last 3 to 10 seconds. Physiologically, orgasmic response is the same whether obtained through masturbation, intercourse, oral stimulation, rubbing stimulation, vibrator stimulation, or manual stimulation. The subjective experience of satisfaction varies, depending on the woman's preferences, partner response, expectations, emotional bond, trust in the relationship, mood, and intensity of stimulation. Each woman develops her own style of being orgasmic. Setting an arbitrary criterion of good or bad types of orgasm is scientifically incorrect and psychologically self-defeating. Multiple orgasms are not better. Focusing on

"G" spot orgasm, deep vaginal orgasm or simultaneous orgasm is the perfect example of making sex a performance goal rather than an experience of shared pleasure. Do not fall into the male trap of pressuring yourself to be orgasmic each time (if not, sex is judged as a failure). You do not need to have the "right" orgasm to prove something to yourself or your partner. Orgasm is a function of being comfortable with and responsible for your sexuality, aware and receptive to stimulation, letting go and allowing yourself to climax. Responsibility includes using your voice to make sexual requests and guide your partner. The male cannot "make" you have an orgasm nor is he responsible for your orgasm. He does need to be caring, cooperative, and sharing.

The Role of Masturbation

Self-exploration, or masturbation, is one of the best ways of learning to become orgasmic. Males have few problems reaching orgasm in part because of their masturbation experiences. The woman who is aware of her arousal and orgasm pattern can transfer this to partner sex. Traditionally, women have been anxious and/or guilty about masturbation. In reality, the majority of women masturbate and frequency actually increases after marriage. Masturbation is not the only route for learning to be orgasmic, but it is a direct, effective, and the most common way to learn about her body, arousal, and orgasm.

Orgasm During Partner Sex

In learning to be orgasmic with a partner, start by examining your assumptions about sexuality. A healthy attitude includes accepting and feeling responsible for your sexuality. The guideline for vital sexuality is to integrate intimacy, non-demand pleasuring, and eroticism. You have a right to be sexually aware, make requests, value eroticism, enjoy arousal, go with the erotic flow, and experience orgasm.

What are your conditions for good sex? How important is being respected by your partner and respecting him? Do you trust your partner and your relationship? Do you feel good about the balance of power in your relationship? Are you happy with the quality and quantity of affection? Are you active and responsive during pleasuring? Are you involved in manual, oral, and rubbing stimulation or do you hold back waiting for intercourse? Can you be orgasmic during erotic, non-intercourse sex or do you withhold or not value that experience? Do you enjoy intercourse as an arousing experience, or are you trying to perform? If you are aroused after your partner has ejaculated, are you comfortable asking for additional stimulation to be orgasmic with afterplay? In examining these issues, be in touch with your sexual values, feelings, and preferences. The majority of women find it easier to be orgasmic with manual, oral, rubbing, or vibrator stimulation than during intercourse. Be aware of blocks which inhibit your natural arousal and orgasmic response.

Medical Interventions as an Additional Resource

Can medical interventions facilitate female desire, arousal, and orgasm? Yes, but not as a substitute for her sexual voice, bridges for desire, taking responsibility for pleasuring and eroticism, and valuing multiple stimulation before and during intercourse. The most effective resources do not require a prescription—use of lubricants and vibrators. What does require seeing a physician (internist or family practice) or a specialist (gynecologist, endocrinologist, or sexual medicine specialist) is conducting a medical history and exam with a special emphasis on evaluating side-effects of medication and the hormonal, vascular and neurological systems. A major cause of sexual dysfunction is side-effects of medications, especially psychiatric and hypertensive medications.

Major medical interventions include testosterone replacement (often in patch form), estrogen supplements, and a Viagra-type drug. None of these directly affects orgasm but all are resources to facilitate the desire and arousal phases of sexual response.

Sherri

Sherri was a thirty-seven-year-old divorcee beginning a new relation-ship with Charles. She was caught in the middle of the sexual revo-lution during her high school years. The learning she received from peers, parents, and church emphasized female virginity and the dou-ble standard. Sherri's older brother had received a very different sex-ual socialization, which gave him permission to experiment without feeling guilty. When Sherri entered college, she was bombarded by the sexual liberation and feminist movements. The transition from the eighteen-year-old conservative and cautious Sherri to the nineteen-year-old experimental and free-wheeling Sherri was extreme and un-settling. She recalls her college years as "sex, drugs, rock music, and liberation." By junior year, she was having orgasms through mastur-bation and, by senior year, orgasms during cunnilingus. After college, she was involved in a series of monogamous dating relationships. Her adult years included times of personal growth intermixed with bouts of depression and lack of direction in her life.

Partly due to insecurity, and partly to peer pressure, she made an unwise marital choice. Sherri was intimidated by her husband ques-tioning her as to why she only had orgasms through oral sex. He de-cided to "help" her by refusing to do cunnilingus so she would have orgasms during intercourse. Sherri felt discounted and disrespected. Her sexual enjoyment decreased and her orgasms disappeared.

After the divorce, Sherri felt negative about herself, men, and sex. She had ambivalent feelings about the dating scene, and in one of her caustic moments, she said single men are either "drunks, neurotics, or gays." For a two-year period she dated only married men because they were considerate, but she tired of the "other woman" role. Sherri was anxious because of her biological clock and desire to have children.

Then Sherri's best friend remarried. After a series of discussions with the friend and new spouse, Sherri decided to date only men she felt comfortable with, attracted to, and trusted. The man would have to value and respect her and be willing to put time and energy into their relationship.

Sherri met Charles while volunteering for a tutoring project. They were friends before they started to date, and they had intercourse three weeks later. The next month Sherri decided to be assertive and talk about sexuality and what she wanted in the relationship.

Initial sexual experiences were okay, but not stimulating. Sherri told Charles that she liked and cared for him and that she wanted this to be a healthy relationship and the sex to be good for both. She told him that in the past six years she had been orgasmic irregularly. Sherri wanted to communicate and make requests so sex could be pleasurable, arousing, and orgasmic. Charles was receptive, but a bit defensive. He too had been divorced, was tired of the dating scene, and looking for a serious relationship. He wanted to be sensitive, yet was afraid she would make sexual demands and view him as a "wimp." Sherri assured him she was looking for an intimate, sharing relationship in which she could make requests and engage in give-and-take. She was not looking for a domineering, demanding relationship.

Charles and Sherri experimented with oral-genital sex. Sherri was pleasantly surprised to find that within three weeks she was responding orgasmically. Sharing, giving, and communication increased emotional intimacy. Anxiety and anger are the major blocks to sexual response. Sherri and Charles dealt with difficult issues outside of the bedroom so these did not interfere with the development of their sexuality.

Charles enjoyed Sherri's orgasms through cunnilingus. For the first time in her life Sherri was multi-orgasmic, which was very arousing for Charles. Rather than pressuring herself to be orgasmic during intercourse, she gave herself permission to experiment and go with her feelings. What proved most effective was Sherri's request for multiple stimulation during intercourse, with her thrusting her pelvis as arousal built and stimulating herself while Charles was thrusting. Sherri learned to be orgasmic during intercourse using multiple stimulation, but preferred oral stimulation as an easier, more intense means of arousal and orgasm. Sherri felt good about her style of being sexually responsive and orgasmic.

Every woman has her own sexual style, so what Sherri enjoyed may or may not be good for you. What is important is being aware of your sexuality and preferences, taking responsibility, being open to sharing and experimenting, and establishing a cooperative, give-and-take relationship.

You are a sexual person who deserves to experience sexual feelings, including orgasm. Each woman has her own sexual style. Do not get hung up on whether you have right or wrong orgasms. Let arousal build and orgasm be the natural culmination of the sexual experience.

First Set of Exercises: Sexual Responsibility

Be the initiator. Design a sexual scenario to promote your comfort, involvement, and arousal. You might begin with a relaxing bath or shower joined by your partner, with holding hands and talking about romantic or erotic feelings, or by receiving a whole body massage. Do what is best for you; it is your sexual show.

If you are easily orgasmic with masturbation, you might stimulate yourself to orgasm with your partner present. Lie comfortably in his arms. Since it is the first time, he could close his eyes so you would not feel self-conscious. Utilize your "orgasm triggers" to carry arousal through to orgasm. This might include moving your pelvis rhythmically, tightening muscles, breathing faster, focusing on a highly charged fantasy, increasing the rhythm of clitoral stimulation, inserting two fingers in your vagina and firmly stimulating the anterior wall, making sounds. Let arousal build and allow it to proceed to climax. Most women find it is easier and more predictable to be orgasmic with masturbation. Being orgasmic with self-stimulation where you feel in control can break down inhibitions about letting go in front of your partner.

If this exercise is not comfortable or you prefer not to be orgasmic with self-stimulation, begin with a partner exercise that emphasizes your responsibility for sexuality. Try a position in which you have freedom to be sexually expressive. Lie on your side so he has easy access to your genitals, on your back with your legs bent so you can move your pelvis, or kneel over him so you can thrust your body toward his hands. Guide your partner, let him know when you are ready for breast and vulva stimulation. Communicating what you want and setting the rhythm of erotic stimulation are crucial. Actively focus on feelings of arousal, heighten them and let go. Allow yourself to express arousal, make noises, breathe as loudly and rapidly as you like. Move your body; ask for breast stimulation; put your hand over his and guide clitoral stimulation; request he put his finger in your vagina and specify how much pressure. Be an active, involved participant and share your arousal.

A sure way to kill arousal is for the man to ask, "Did you come?" Orgasm is not an isolated goal. The woman can share how aroused or high she felt and the sensations and stimulation she valued. She can request additional stimulation or suggest scenarios and positions to explore in subsequent exercises. If you attain orgasm, that's great. You can share this or discuss it another time. If you do not, take what you have learned and continue to increase your pleasure, stimulation and arousal.

Second Set of Exercises: Multiple Stimulation

There are two major strategies for building arousal to orgasm: 1) focusing on multiple stimulation to heighten arousal and orgasm, and 2) becoming comfortable with expressing yourself, letting go and using "orgasm triggers." This exercise incorporates both strategies. There is a ban on intercourse, but no prohibition on the variety and type of stimulation you can request and utilize. Less than 5 percent of women experience their first orgasm during intercourse. Most have first orgasm via masturbation, oral stimulation, manual stimulation, vibrator stimulation or rubbing against your partner.

Choose the pleasuring position(s) in which you can be most expressive. Set the rhythm of sensual and erotic stimulation. Take your time; allow yourself to be selfish, set the pace that is best for you. Instead of trying to second-guess or worry if your partner is bored or frustrated, realize that he is learning that a receptive, responsive partner is the best aphrodisiac. Tell him when to begin genital stimulation and how you like your genitals touched. Many women prefer beginning with light, teasing breast stroking; others prefer oral stimulation of the areola; others choose rhythmic stroking of the vulva with a focus on the labia; others enjoy touching from the mons to the clitoral shaft; still others prefer stimulation around the perineum and up to the labia. What is your preferred pattern? Share this with your partner.

Do you prefer to intermix non-genital and genital stimulation or do you respond to focused erotic stimulation? Some women find oral breast stimulation and manual clitoral stimulation, combined with sexual fantasy, a great combination. For others having the vulva orally stimulated and moving the pelvis in rhythm with arousal while stroking the partner's penis is the right combination. For others, a combination of clitoral shaft and manual stimulation of the anterior wall of the vagina while watching an erotic video is most arousing. Some find combining clitoral stimulation with anal stimulation while the partner verbalizes a sexually explicit fantasy best allows them to let go and be orgasmic. Some women prefer one continuous focused stimulation rather than multiple stimulation. Each woman and couple develop their particular styles of sharing eroticism, arousal and coming to orgasm. Share arousal and orgasm "with" your partner rather than looking to him to "make" you have an orgasm. Do not try to "will" or "force" an orgasm.

What thoughts, actions, or sensations serve as "orgasm triggers"? Some women let go with a specific fantasy, increase rhythm of pelvic thrusting, touch themselves in special ways, focus on breathing, or verbalize that they are "going to come." Others increase stimulation of their partner and as his arousal builds so does hers. Are there orgasm triggers you have not shared because of embarrassment, lack of assertiveness, or the feeling that it's not proper? It is perfectly proper and acceptable to share special turn-ons and orgasm triggers. This is the time to be assertive; so share your erotic preferences and let go.

Some women know that if they touch themselves or use vibrator stimulation in addition to partner stimulation, they will be orgasmic. Yet they refrain from doing so because they think it is not "right" and are afraid their partner will be offended because it seems "out of control" or "kinky." Being orgasmic in front of your partner is a breakthrough. Instead of inhibiting yourself by saying "it's not the right way," give yourself permission to engage in highly erotic stimulation and utilize orgasm triggers. Most couples are pleasantly surprised that when the walls of inhibition and embarrassment fall down, a host of alternatives for further experimentation and sharing open up.

The experience need not end at the point of orgasm (yours or his). You can pleasure your partner and help him be orgasmic. Whether either or both have been orgasmic, afterplay is an integral part of the sexual experience. Come down together, not with the burden of whether you succeeded or failed, but sharing what you learned about multiple stimulation, orgasm triggers, special turn-ons, being expressive, and letting go. Tell him what you would like to experiment with next time.

Third Set of Exercises:
Multiple Stimulation During Intercourse

Approximately 55 to 65 percent of women experience orgasm during intercourse. Does this mean 35 to 45 percent of women are dysfunctional? Not at all. Being orgasmic in erotic, non-intercourse sex is a normal, healthy expression of female sexuality. Most women prefer to be orgasmic during non-intercourse sex rather than during intercourse. Some women prefer to be orgasmic during intercourse; others prefer to be orgasmic with manual, rubbing, or oral stimulation (including those who can be orgasmic during intercourse). There is no "one right" pattern.

Intercourse can be a pleasurable, shared experience whether it results in orgasm or not. This exercise focuses on increasing involvement, pleasure and arousal during intercourse. If it increases orgasmic response, so much the better, but orgasm during intercourse is not the main goal. The focus is on increasing eroticism, arousal, and multiple stimulation during intercourse.

Women have traditionally viewed intercourse as the man's domain. In this exercise, however, she initiates intercourse and chooses the position she finds most pleasurable. A common pitfall is for her to establish a rhythm of arousal during pleasuring and then relinquish it when intercourse begins. Another common trap is the cessation of multiple stimulation with intercourse. In this exercise she sets the coital rhythm, and she and her partner engage in multiple stimulation throughout intercourse.

Do you want to initiate touching or would you like your partner to? Whoever initiates, it is she who determines when to begin intercourse. Do not start intercourse at the first sign of arousal. Continue stimulation and allow arousal to build. Be aware of multiple stimulation techniques which add to arousal and continue using them throughout intercourse. Guide your partner's penis into you. After all, you are the world's expert on your vagina. Try intercourse in the woman-on-top or another position that gives you freedom of movement and expression. Variations of side, rear-entry, and sitting positions are preferred alternatives.

What is your favorite thrusting movement? In-out, circular, or up–down? Set the speed and rhythm which facilitates sexual expression. What additional stimulation do you enjoy during intercourse? Should he stroke your breasts, or with your hands massaging the clitoris, should his two fingers stimulate your anal area? Should you stroke his chest, kiss, verbalize erotic fantasies, use a vibrator for simultaneous clitoral stimulation, scratch his back? Clearly, directly, and assertively request what you want. Do not be embarrassed to utilize fantasies to increase arousal; erotic fantasies are the most common form of multiple stimulation. Do what increases involvement, eroticism and arousal during intercourse. If you like, you could interrupt intercourse, use manual or oral stimulation to heighten arousal, then resume intercourse in a different position, continuing with multiple stimulation.

If you reach orgasm, how do you feel? Some women really enjoy the sensations, while others are disappointed because it is not as physiologically intense as they had hoped. If you are not orgasmic during intercourse, that's perfectly normal. Many, in fact most, women find it easier to be orgasmic during non-intercourse sex. Be aware of positions and techniques which allow you to be an involved, aroused intercourse partner.

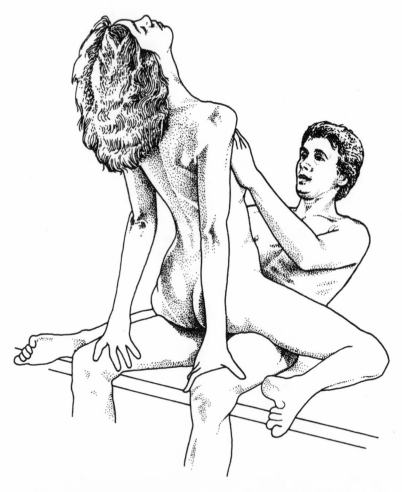

Breast stimulation of female in superior intercourse position, to maximize the pleasure of her sexual experience.

Fourth Set of Exercises:
Being Responsible for Your Orgasm

You have experimented with pleasuring and intercourse positions, voicing your sexual preferences, using multiple stimulation, being active during pleasuring and intercourse, and making specific requests. This exercise asks you to develop your favorite arousal and orgasm scenario.

You are the expert on your sexuality. You are responsible for your comfort, desire, pleasure, arousal, and orgasm. This responsibility cannot be assumed by your partner or by exercises. Design your own exercise (sexual scenario) for eroticism, arousal, and orgasm.

Start from the beginning: What are your conditions for sexual comfort and desire? Who initiates? When? Where? What is most important about your partner's attitudes, behavior, and feelings? What can he do to enhance your sexual receptiveness and responsiveness?

Once comfort is established, how can you increase pleasure? Do you like stimulation to be slow and tender, teasing and seductive, or erotic and genitally focused? Do you like romantic music, your partner verbalizing sexual feelings, the use of pictures or videos, reading erotic fantasies? Do you want to be pleasured or do you prefer mutual stimulation? Do you like lying in bed, standing in front of a mirror, kneeling facing each other in front of the fireplace, being sexual in the shower? Are there special pleasuring positions and turn-ons which facilitate arousal?

What initiatives or requests will build arousal? Do you respond to special stimulation—a vibrator, touching yourself, simultaneous oral and anal simulation, breast and clitoral stimulation, clitoral and vaginal stimulation? Is your partner's arousal vital to your arousal? Feel free to request and guide. Are you most responsive to manual, oral, vibrator, rubbing or intercourse stimulation? Focus on and enjoy arousal, allowing it to flow and build.

What are your orgasm triggers and how expressive are you during orgasm? Do you make sounds and move or just allow your body to let go? Do you focus on a single form of stimulation or do you prefer multiple stimulation? Do you actively move toward orgasm or let arousal build and sweep you to orgasm? Do you feel free to utilize triggers? Maximize your expressiveness and satisfaction.

Closing Thoughts

Orgasm is not the ultimate test of sexual satisfaction, nor is it a measure of femininity. It is a natural psychophysiological response to involved, effective sexual stimulation that causes high levels of arousal to naturally culminate in orgasm. Each woman has her own style of being orgasmic. Enjoy orgasm as a way of sharing an intimate sexual experience that validates you as a sexual woman and enhances your sexual relationship.

17

Learning Ejaculatory Control

Myths about male sexual performance are among the most powerful negative influences on a couple's sexual functioning. It was once believed that the more masculine you were, the faster you ejaculated. The new myth would prove masculinity with intercourse that lasts for half an hour without ejaculation. The majority of adolescent and young adult males begin as early ejaculators. Most men, as they gain experience, do learn ejaculatory control. However, approximately three in ten males have difficulty with early ejaculation. The average time for intercourse, from intromission to ejaculation, is between two and seven minutes. The great majority of males ejaculate in less than ten minutes.

Early Ejaculation

There is much confusion as to what early ejaculation is. Some people define it in terms of time (thirty seconds after intromission), some in terms of activity (fewer than ten strokes), some in terms of whether the woman is orgasmic during intercourse (an extremely poor criterion). Masters and Johnson stated that if the woman is normally orgasmic during intercourse, early ejaculation occurs if the man ejaculates before the woman's orgasm in 50 percent of intercourse encounters. These definitions are too arbitrary and performance-oriented. A more reasonable approach is that if the couple is making good use of non-genital and genital pleasuring, and the man's ejaculation is earlier than desired and interferes with pleasure, then there is a reason to improve ejaculatory control. The typical lovemaking experience involves fifteen to forty-five minutes, of which two to seven minutes is engaged in intercourse.

Many males could benefit from training in ejaculatory control. Instead of viewing early ejaculation as a major problem that makes the man inadequate or causes the woman to feel her sexual needs are being ignored, think of ejaculatory control as a skill the couple—not just the male—can learn in order to enhance mutual sexual satisfaction.

How Early Ejaculation Develops

Males learn early ejaculation from a host of cultural and personal experiences. Adolescent masturbation is very penis-oriented and orgasm-oriented, so early ejaculation is over-learned. The male's first intercourse might take place in the back seat of a car in a hurried, unplanned way, on a couch in the woman's house with the fear her parents might discover him, or with a prostitute who applies pressure to "hurry up and get it over with." These experiences have the common denominator of high sexual excitement mixed with anxiety, with a pressure to perform rapidly. The male is more concerned with proving himself and reaching orgasm than enjoying his partner's pleasure or his pleasure with touching and sensual feelings. In learning ejaculatory control, he breaks the association between high anxiety and high arousal and learns to enjoy a range of sexual stimulation. He needs to prolong arousal and learns to associate arousal with awareness and pleasure.

Some men believe ejaculating rapidly shows how masculine and sexually assured they are. The male with this mind-set does not see intercourse as a mutual act, but as something the male does to the female, her needs and desires being unimportant. Lack of sexual knowledge, masturbatory experiences that emphasize coming as fast as possible, early experiences pairing sexual excitement with anxiety, a habit pattern of rapid ejaculation, and not accepting sexuality as a mutual experience leads to the man becoming an early ejaculator.

Learning Ejaculatory Control

Whatever the origin of early ejaculation, you can learn ejaculatory control. In the optimal situation, the partners work cooperatively, for indeed the woman's role is highly important. Learning ejaculatory control is a couple task.

Ejaculatory exercises are built upon the solid foundation of non-genital and genital pleasuring. You will be both giving and receiving pleasure as well as learning specific skills. Ejaculatory control is not about the man performing up to a standard or proving he can give the woman an orgasm during intercourse, but about developing a mutually satisfying couple style that includes pleasure-oriented intercourse.

Traps and Distractions

A man with a history of early ejaculation frequently falls into psychological traps. He feels negative about ejaculation and apologizes for himself sexually. Rather than enjoying orgasm, he mentally kicks himself for coming too fast. This does not in any way help his ejaculatory control. Sometimes he even tries to avoid sex—which is counter-productive because the less regular the sexual interaction, the more likely his ejaculation will be rapid.

Another trap involves distractions. Males often try various distraction techniques in their usually vain effort to postpone ejaculation during intercourse, They think of the bills they owe, a TV program, or their mother-in-law. They attempt physical distractions such as clenching a fist, biting a lip, or pinching themselves. Other males put an anesthetizing cream on the glans of the penis or wear two or three condoms—all misguided counter-productive techniques. In attempting to control orgasm, the man distracts himself from the stimulation of touch, arousal, and intercourse. He is tuning out sexual feelings. In the worst case, he turns himself off so he has difficulty maintaining his arousal and erection. As a result, his partner feels neglected or rejected by his lack of involvement and excitement. This can lead to a decline in her arousal and negative feelings about their relationship. Distracting strategies are based on the premise that it is solely the male's responsibility to control his ejaculation, and the best way to do this is to avoid arousal and penile stimulation. That is false. Distracting strategies add to sexual and relationship problems. Treatment of ejaculatory control is counter-intuitive, the emphasis is on increasing penile stimulation, not avoiding arousal and stimulation.

Bernie and Cindy

Bernie and Cindy had been married eight years. Cindy had not raised the issue of early ejaculation until four months before they sought out a therapist. Bernie had become upset and defensive as well as obsessed with solving the problem. During the ensuing four months Bernie and Cindy's sexual experiences became a command performance in which the goal was for Cindy to reach orgasm first (during intercourse). It was a crucial test of manhood to "hold out" until she had an orgasm. Instead, Cindy stopped having orgasms of any kind and Bernie was reaching orgasm shortly after intromission. This was not an intimate, sharing experience. Theirs was a dispirited relationship sinking under the weight of performance pressure.

Ejaculatory control is gradually learned by a couple working in a cooperative manner. Bernie was being his own worst enemy and turning Cindy off. The first priority was to return pleasure and intimacy to their sexual relationship. Bernie had misinterpreted Cindy's comments as meaning that he was a terrible lover. With the intervention of the therapist, Bernie was able to understand that Cindy valued their marriage and saw him as a loving, attractive person. Her request was for Bernie to be a more sensitive, slower lover. Cindy has a variable arousal and orgasmic pattern; she enjoys being orgasmic during manual and oral stimulation as well as intercourse. Intercourse would be enhanced for her by better ejaculatory control on Bernie's part, but Cindy was not demanding perfect performance. Bernie needed to realize that prolonging intercourse would be of value for him. He was learning ejaculatory control for himself and the relationship, not to perform for Cindy. With this new attitude and couple commitment learning ejaculatory control became easier for Bernie.

Ejaculatory control exercises can at times be tedious, but if the couple are cooperative and communicating, it can be enjoyable. Some women complain the stop-start exercises are boring and they feel like a marionette who stops on command. Cindy wanted to feel that she was an integral part of the experience and that her feelings and needs were important. As a bonus, Cindy and Bernie expanded their repertoire of pleasuring and erotic techniques. Both learned to be sexually assertive, to express feelings, and enjoy flexible, variable sexual expression.

Shared Responsibility

Learning ejaculatory control employs the one-two combination of the male increasing awareness and the couple working as an intimate team. The best way to develop ejaculatory control is through the couple's active participation and commitment. The most successful strategy increases comfort, builds awareness of penile sensations, and teaches ejaculatory control skills. It also requires patience and persistence. You will learn two key skills—to identify the point of ejaculatory inevitability and to increase the time from arousal to ejaculation.

Sexual arousal is a naturally occurring, voluntary response up to the point of ejaculatory inevitability. At this point, ejaculation becomes an involuntary response, i.e., the male will ejaculate even if he tries to stop it. If stimulation ceases *before* the point of ejaculatory inevitability, this retards the urge to ejaculate. The male gradually learns to maintain sexual arousal without going to the point of ejaculatory inevitability. When he is able to enjoy arousal during prolonged intercourse (five to ten minutes), the couple has learned ejaculatory control and will enjoy more satisfying intercourse.

A more conventional procedure is the "squeeze technique." Though effective, many people find it objectionable because it is too mechanical. You will be using the "start–stop" technique.

Medication as a Resource

There is a growing trend to use medication, either at a low dose continuously or a moderate dose two hours before intercourse, to treat ejaculatory control. This involves antidepressant medication and does delay ejaculation for the majority of men. However, effectiveness requires continual use of the medication; if you stop, the early ejaculation returns and sometimes even more severely. Although men find taking a "magic pill" to solve the early ejaculation problem more inviting than working with their partner, we do not advocate this approach.

If you choose to use medication, the preferred strategy is to use medication as an additional resource in conjunction with the ejaculatory control exercises. A major strategy is to slow down the entire sexual process, including intercourse. As comfort and confidence with ejaculatory control increases, you can gradually decrease your dependence on medication.

First Set of Exercises: Stop–Start

Talk about positive feelings and experiences with non-genital and genital pleasuring. You are learning to give and receive sexual feedback.

Start with mutual pleasuring. Then arrange yourselves in a position where the female partner leans back comfortably with her back supported by a pillow or cushion against the bed's headboard. The male positions his body between her spread legs, lying on his back facing her and with his legs bent and lying outside her thighs. Vary positioning until you feel comfortable.

The woman begins massaging her partner's chest, slowly and naturally, working down to his genitals. As responsiveness and arousal increase, he will naturally get an erection. A few moments after his erection begins, she stops penile stimulation.

After stimulation ceases, he loses both the urge to ejaculate and the rigidity of his erection—perhaps half of it. This happens because the cessation of genital stimulation interrupts blood flow to the penis. She ceases stimulation well before he has the urge to ejaculate. This provides practice in using the stop-start technique.

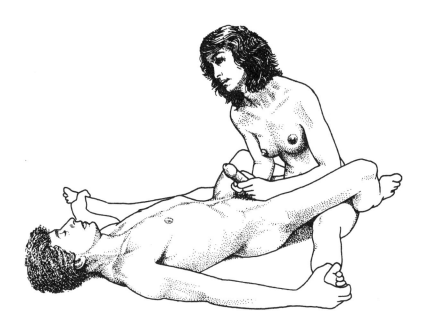

Manual penile stimulation in the practice of stop-start exercises for ejaculatory control.

After thirty to sixty seconds, the woman returns to sexual fondling and manual stimulation. She need not concentrate all her time on the penis. She can massage the man's stomach, teasingly play with his testicles, run her fingers along his inner thighs, and at the same time make the touching enjoyable and sensuous for herself. Responding to sensual and sexual feelings, the male allows arousal to build. If he does not regain an erection, neither partner should worry—simply enjoy sensual feelings. For many couples, this is their first experience with the physiologically normal process of waxing and waning erections. Most males are conditioned to go to orgasm on their first erection.

Previously, the man avoided focusing on penile sensations because he was afraid he would become too excited and ejaculate. In this exercise, he focuses on and accepts erotic, arousing feelings. Awareness of sexual sensations allows him to become a better discriminator of his excitement, especially as he approaches the point of ejaculatory inevitability. Identifying the sexual feelings that precede the point of inevitability is a crucial step in learning ejaculatory control.

This exercise enables the couple to develop a mutually agreed-upon communication system to signal when to stop penile stimulation. Some common signals are his saying "now," raising one hand, saying "stop," or tapping her hand. The man signals *before* he reaches the point of ejaculatory inevitability, and she stops penile stimulation immediately.

Use the stop-start technique for at least ten minutes. There are usually at least three stops. For practice, she can stop early in the arousal cycle and again after he has had an erection for a minute. If at any point he feels that he is approaching the point of inevitability, he signals her *immediately* so she can stop. If he does ejaculate, neither partner need feel upset or guilty. Enjoy the ejaculation. Making a mistake and ejaculating early is a normal part of the learning process.

When you feel comfortable with the concepts of ejaculatory control and have utilized the stop-start technique at least three times, you have done well. The male may request continued manual stimulation to ejaculation. At this point, too, his partner deserves to be the recipient of pleasuring. She can guide him in the type of pleasuring she finds particularly sensual or sexually arousing. He is actively involved in giving pleasure and enjoying her responsiveness.

Get dressed and over a drink or coffee share your feelings about the stop-start technique. First discuss what you enjoyed and valued. Then be honest in sharing negative feelings. Many couples report that stopping feels awkward or clinical. Some men report embarrassment at being the center of attention. Some women feel they are playing the role of sexual servant. Many couples feel funny about prohibiting intercourse and using manual sex to orgasm. If you have negative feelings, air them with the partner listening respectfully. You can consider alterations which will increase comfort, but do not stop the ejaculatory control focus. Be aware that learning ejaculatory control is a process which takes practice, feedback, and commitment.

Second Set of Exercises: Continued Practice

Start with affectionate, playful, non-demand pleasuring, then change to the ejaculatory control position. The man should be comfortable, lying on his back with legs stretched out so that the woman has full access to his genitals.

The woman begins by directly massaging and caressing the penis in the most stimulating manner possible, bringing the man close to the point of ejaculatory inevitability. She should stroke the penis with one hand and, simultaneously, touch the testicles in a teasing manner, caress his inner thighs or run her fingers over his pubic hair. As he approaches the point of inevitability, he should signal her to stop stimulation. During the thirty- to sixty-second break he will lose the urge to ejaculate and partially lose his erection.

Since he is learning to discriminate the point of ejaculatory inevitability, the man will probably signal late at least once and will ejaculate. Do not worry; this is natural and important in learning discrimination. Males who are concurrently practicing ejaculatory control via masturbation exercises realize they need continued practice to discriminate the point of ejaculatory inevitability and gradually increase confidence with prolonged stimulation. Enjoy ejaculation rather than being angry or disappointed. The woman can accept this rather than feel frustrated with her partner or herself. Learning ejaculatory control takes practice, mistakes, feedback, cooperation and persistence. When the male ejaculates, proceed to female pleasuring. There is no reason for sex to end because he ejaculates. If he is interested and desires to, you can return to penile stimulation and the stop-start procedure after a twenty to thirty minute break.

Continue stimulation for at least ten minutes. Do this even if you must stop ten times! Wait thirty to sixty seconds and begin restimulation when the male reports that he no longer feels the urge to ejaculate. Use a variety of stimulation techniques. Be aware of and enjoy his responsiveness. Reverse roles and allow the woman to enjoy and respond to pleasure, with the man utilizing his personal style of pleasuring and enjoying her arousal to orgasm if she wishes. He can be orgasmic with her stimulation or during intercourse (at this point, do not expect intercourse to be prolonged).

Repeat this exercise at least twice. In subsequent experiences, use K-Y jelly or a hypoallergenic lotion (abalone oil, Johnson's Baby Oil, scented lotion from Crabtree and Evelyn) to lubricate the penis. The sensations are similar to those during intercourse when the penis is moving inside her lubricated vagina. An alternative is oral (fellatio) stimulation. The lubrication from licking and sucking and the high levels of arousal generated facilitates practice in ejaculatory control. Another stimulation technique is for the woman to use her breasts. She can begin by rubbing his penis around each breast in a gentle, sensuous manner and then proceeding to rhythmic, erotic thrusting on the breast. She can put his penis in the crevice between the breasts. If she has large breasts, bring the breasts together and move them while encircling the penis. This simulates movement of the vagina during intercourse.

When he feels the urge to ejaculate, she immediately stops stimulation. Be sure that the man can discriminate and identify the point of ejaculatory inevitability and that the woman uses the stop-start technique to retard the urge to ejaculate. He can focus on, and allow himself to enjoy, the feelings in his penis (and entire body) at high levels of arousal. It is important both are comfortable and confident with these skills before moving to intravaginal exercises. When he is comfortable and confident with the extravaginal ejaculatory control process, it is easier to generalize ejaculatory control to intercourse.

Third Set of Exercises: Quiet Vagina

Now that you have learned the basic techniques of ejaculatory control, utilize them during intercourse. The best intercourse position for practice is female-on-top. This position is good both for ejaculatory control and for increasing female initiative, activity and responsivity. The male lies on his back, his legs stretched out against the bed. The woman lies over him with her knees at his chest so her vulva is adjacent to his genital area. She rests her buttocks on his thighs. From this position she can manually stimulate his penis as well as rub it around her clitoris, labia, and vaginal introitus.

After utilizing the stop-start technique, restimulate the penis. When he becomes erect, she guides his penis (her hand on it) by placing the penis in at about a forty-five degree angle and sliding back. After intromission, remain still; just allow the penis to remain in the vagina. This is called the "quiet vagina" exercise. The man makes no movement; he simply enjoys the feeling of intravaginal containment. He can focus on the warm, sensual feelings of his penis being contained in her vagina. Some women find this arousing, others do not. Stay with and accept the feelings; avoid thrusting. She moves slowly and nondemandingly; use only enough movement to insure he maintains penile sensations.

If at any point the man feels himself approaching the point of ejaculatory inevitability, he should signal his partner to stop movement. If that is not enough to retard arousal, he can ask her to disengage from intercourse and lie next to him. Allow "quiet vagina" intercourse to proceed for ten to fifteen minutes. Feel free to use the stop-start technique as often as needed. Repeat the "quiet vagina" exercise at least once at a later time.

It is preferable to use the stop-start technique at least three times during intercourse. If the man does ejaculate (whether within the vagina or extravaginally), accept and enjoy it. You are learning to discriminate the point of ejaculatory inevitability as well as to elongate the time between arousal and ejaculation. This takes practice, supportive feedback, and refining ejaculatory control skills.

In the female-on-top position, you have the advantage of mutual pleasuring. The man can massage and touch his partner during intercourse. She can accept and enjoy feelings of sensuality and arousal. End the exercise by continuing intercourse to orgasm, using slow thrusting.

Repeat this set of exercises until you are comfortable and confident with ejaculatory control in the female-on-top intercourse position. The woman should gradually increase coital thrusting and experiment with in-out, up-down, and circular movements. In subsequent experiences, the man can control thrusting, beginning with slow, long movements. Most couples find rapid, in-out, short strokes the most difficult movement for ejaculatory control. Talk about feelings of progress and pleasure as you continue to work together, enhance ejaculatory control, and enjoy the entire sexual experience.

Fourth Set of Exercises: Active Intercourse

This set of exercises involves the side by side position. The woman can gently stroke the man's face and chest, move to manual penile stimulation, and rub his penis around her clitoris, labia, and vagina. After intromission, she can initiate gentle, slow, long thrusting. When he feels an urge to ejaculate, he signals and coital movement should stop. After the urge to ejaculate decreases, she returns to slow, sensuous thrusting. If he is having difficulty maintaining ejaculatory control, temporarily disengage from intercourse.

Many couples find intromission easier by beginning in the man or woman on top position and then rolling into the side-by-side position. Allow the second intromission to be comfortable and gradual with minimal thrusting. Then engage in thrusting controlled by the woman, while the man focuses on arousal and penile sensations. As he approaches the point of ejaculatory inevitability, he should signal her to stop stimulation, but stay in this intercourse position. As with the other exercises, you are encouraged to repeat this process; each repetition increases confidence. Remember, ejaculatory control is learned gradually and requires practice and feedback. As you become comfortable, slow or vary the rhythm of thrusting rather than totally stopping. Most couples require three to six months to develop comfort and confidence with ejaculatory control during intercourse.

The next steps are:

1. The man initiates slow, nondemand thrusting.
2. The woman initiates more rapid, involving thrusting.
3. The man initiates more rapid, involving thrusting.

In practicing each step, remember to use the stop-start technique as necessary. When early ejaculation occurs, accept and enjoy it. Remember, sexual interaction need not end because the man has ejaculated.

At each step try for five to seven minutes of intravaginal containment without ejaculation; even if you use the stop-start technique many times. Repeat each step at least twice, and more, if you want. As comfort and confidence build, you will need to use the stop-start technique less.

Begin using a variant of the stop-start technique: slowing the rhythm of coital movement as you approach the point of ejaculatory inevitability. When the urge to ejaculate disappears, return to active thrusting.

When you have maintained ejaculatory control for five to seven minutes, you can proceed to ejaculation. The decision to complete intercourse is a mutual one; do not feel pressure to make each intercourse a perfect experience. Allow yourselves to enjoy intercourse and orgasm. Share the warm, intimate feelings of afterplay.

Sex does not end with the man's ejaculation. Many women enjoy manual or rubbing stimulation after intercourse—either for arousal and orgasm or to share physical closeness. Sharing feelings about the sexual experience is important. Realize how far you have come, not only in learning ejaculatory control but becoming an intimate, loving couple.

Guidelines—Learning Ejaculatory Control

These guidelines are used to promote ejaculatory control and prevent relapse.

1. Early ejaculation is the most frequent male sexual problem. The majority of adolescents and young adults begin as early ejaculators. Thirty percent of adult males complain of early ejaculation.

2. "Do it yourself" techniques to reduce arousal (biting your lip, focusing on non-sexual thoughts such as how much money you owe, using two condoms or a penile desensitizing cream) do not help in gaining ejaculatory control. By reducing arousal, these techniques can cause erectile dysfunction.

3. Learning ejaculatory control involves identifying the point of ejaculatory inevitability (after which ejaculation is no longer a voluntary function) and maintaining awareness at high levels of arousal.

4. Ejaculatory control can be learned both through self-stimulation and partner stimulation. Use self-stimulation to develop awareness, to increase comfort, and to learn skills. This builds confidence and motivation in partner sex. Ejaculatory control during partner sex, especially intercourse, is complex and challenging.

5. The strategy in learning ejaculatory control is counter-intuitive. Increase comfort, awareness, and stimulation; do not decrease stimulation or arousal.

6. The most effective technique is "stop-start." The man signals his partner to stop stimulation as he approaches the point of inevitability. Stimulation stops for thirty to sixty seconds, until he no longer feels the need to ejaculate. The couple then resumes stimulation. Most couples prefer this rather than the traditional "squeeze" technique, which can be awkward and mechanical.

7. The stop-start technique is used first with manual stimulation, then oral stimulation, and before and during intercourse. Learn-

ing ejaculatory control is a gradual process requiring practice, feedback, and persistence.

8. Realistic expectations and goals are crucial. The typical love-making experience extends from fifteen to forty-five minutes, of which two to seven minutes involve intercourse. Contrary to male bragging and media myths, intercourse seldom lasts longer than ten minutes.

9. Only one in four women have the same response pattern as men, i.e. a single orgasm during intercourse. One in three orgasmic women are never orgasmic during intercourse. Improved ejaculatory control increases pleasure and eroticism for the man and couple. The goal of ejaculatory control is *not* to guarantee the woman has an orgasm during intercourse.

10. The stop-start technique is used during intercourse. Initially, the man stops movement or withdraws. As awareness and confidence increase, the strategy is to use slower or circular thrusting.

11. Typically, ejaculatory control exercises during intercourse begin with the woman on top position using minimal movement (the quiet vagina exercise). She guides intromission and controls thrusting.

12. With continued practice, other intercourse positions are added. Utilize longer, slower thrusting or circular thrusting. Alternate which partner controls the thrusting. Ejaculatory control is most difficult in the man on top position with short, rapid thrusting.

13. Try to maintain ejaculatory control for ten minutes with non-intercourse stimulation (self-stimulation and partner manual or oral stimulation). Try to maintain ejaculatory control with four to seven minutes of intercourse stimulation.

14. When you ejaculate, whether rapidly or voluntarily, enjoy the feelings and sensations, do not be upset or angry. "Beating up" on yourself does not facilitate ejaculatory control.

15. Feelings and sensations of orgasm begin at the point of ejaculatory inevitability and last three to ten seconds.

16. The woman's emotional and sexual feelings are very important. Her role is an intimate, involved partner. The man can pleasure her to arousal and orgasm with manual, oral, rubbing, or vibrator

stimulation. Most women prefer this after the ejaculatory control exercise, but some prefer it before. Sex need not end when the man ejaculates.

17. Some men prefer to use medication, either at a low dose continuously or a moderate dose two hours before intercourse, to promote ejaculatory control. Anti-depressant medications are the most commonly used and are effective for the majority of men. However, success is dependent on remaining on medication.

18. The preferred strategy is to use medication as an additional resource. Practice ejaculatory control exercises while taking medication and then gradually eliminate medication.

19. Remember, do not try to reduce stimulation or feeling "turned on." You do not want to develop an arousal problem, i.e. erectile dysfunction. Focus on comfort, awareness, pleasure, and enjoying arousal without moving rapidly to ejaculation.

20. Sexuality is about giving and receiving pleasure, not a perfect performance. Enjoy and share the entire sexual experience—intimacy, pleasure, eroticism, arousal, intercourse, and afterplay.

Closing Thoughts

Learning ejaculatory control is like learning any skill. It is a gradual process requiring feedback and refining techniques. Practice the last set of exercises at least a couple of weeks before moving on to other intercourse positions. Male-on-top is the most difficult intercourse position for ejaculatory control. One of the best for ejaculatory control and mutual sexual responsiveness is the lateral coital position (refer to the third intercourse exercise in Chapter 9). Use slower thrusting and stop-start techniques for a year or more. It is especially important to utilize these when you have intercourse after a break of a week or more. Maintain open communication as you progress in feeling comfortable and confident (not performing to a perfect standard) with ejaculatory control. Integrate non-genital sensual touching, genital pleasuring, intercourse, and afterplay into your couple sexual style.

18

Arousal and Erections

Far too much of a man's self-esteem and sense of masculinity is tied to his penis. Fear of erectile dysfunction (commonly called "impotence" or "not getting it up") is among the greatest of all male fears. A well-hidden fact of male sexuality is that by age forty 90 percent of men have experienced on at least one occasion a problem either obtaining or maintaining an erection sufficient for intercourse. Man's most feared experience is, in fact, an almost universal one. Males are notorious liars and braggarts about sexual prowess. They adamantly deny sexual doubts or difficulties. Males suffer discomfort and intimidation from the myth-based cultural expectation that "a real man is able and willing to have sex with any woman, at any time, in any situation." This puts a tremendous performance pressure on the man—and his penis.

The majority of erectile dysfunction is caused primarily by psychological or relationship problems rather than physical or medical factors. This is especially true for males under fifty. An erection involves increased blood flow to the penis (vasocongestion) which fills the tissues and increases the size of the penis. As arousal builds, rigidity (hardness) increases. These functions depend on a healthy neurological system.

The hormonal, vascular and neurological systems must be functional for adequate erectile response. Common physical causes of erectile dysfunction include alcoholism, uncontrolled diabetes, prostatectomy surgery, side effects from hypertensive or psychiatric medications, spinal cord injury, and chronic illness. As the male ages, his hormonal, vascular, and neurological systems function at lower levels of efficacy. Thus, he is more vulnerable to anticipatory and performance anxiety. A fifty-year-old man is not the easy, automatic, autonomous sexual athlete he was at twenty. His sexual response becomes less predictable and more variable. Psychological, intimacy, and sexual technique factors become more important with aging (though they are of importance for males of all ages). If you have questions about physical or medical aspects of your sexual functioning, the best person to consult is a urologist. Although not typically considered a male sex doctor, the urologist cares for men much the way a gynecologist does for women. Be sure the urologist is interested in doing a comprehensive assessment, and not promoting Viagra, testosterone, penile injections, or an external pump.

The major causes of erectile problems are performance anxiety and distraction from the erotic flow. The male is so concerned with proving himself or performing up to perfect, fantasy expectations that he becomes anxious. This interferes with sexual responsivity and arousal. Anxiety is physiologically incompatible with feelings of sensuality and eroticism. When the man experiences anticipatory or performance anxiety, worry or tension, erections are inhibited.

Another crucial factor is the male sexual transition that comes with aging. Young males learn that erections are easy, automatic, predictable and autonomous (needing nothing from the woman). In a male's thirties and forties, however, the hormonal, vascular and neurologic systems change. Sexuality becomes a function of receptiveness and responsiveness to partner stimulation. Sex becomes a cooperative, interactive experience. As the man enters his fifties, side effects of medications, stress, and health problems can effect a now more vulnerable arousal system. Intimacy, pleasuring, and erotic scenarios become ever more important in facilitating arousal and erection.

Another cause of erection problems is negative reactions such as guilt, anger, depression, or ambivalence. If either partner feels negative emotions in regard to sexuality, this inhibits responsiveness and arousal—and therefore erections.

In order to increase pleasure and eroticism, no matter what the interfering factors, the couple should strive to develop a cooperative, sharing, sexual relationship. Lack of arousal and erection is not the problem of the man alone; it is best considered a couple issue. Regaining comfort and confidence with arousal and erections is the couple's task. In helping her partner increase sexual responsiveness, a woman can learn to accept and enjoy her sexuality. Her sexual responsiveness and arousal is a friend to the couple's relationship. Each partner contributes to the erotic flow of their sexuality, and each should follow and extend the give-to-get pleasuring guideline. A crucial step is to affirm their desire to work together to increase feelings of arousal and revitalize their sexual relationship.

The Self-Defeating Cycle of Erectile Failure

You cannot *will* an erection. You cannot produce an erection by making demands, whether by self-pressure or partner pressure. The man who has had difficulty getting or maintaining an erection concentrates on his penis and attempts to force an erection (which is self-defeating). The more he works at achieving erection, the less success he will have. Erection is a natural result of involvement, receptivity to sensual and erotic stimulation, and enjoyment of your own and partner's subjective arousal. Erection is not something to be striven for. When the male focuses attention on his penis, he takes himself out of the erotic flow and plays the role of spectator. Rather than being involved with his partner's feelings and the enjoyment of pleasuring and eroticism, the spectator focuses on the state of his penis. Instead of being an active, giving sexual partner—which facilitates arousal and erection—he is a passive, anxious observer of his penis. Sex is not a spectator sport where you lie back and have your performance judged. When sex and performance are linked together, you are halfway to having a dysfunction. The positive association is between sex and pleasure, the give and take process of sharing pleasure, eroticism, and arousal.

Active Involvement

The best way for the couple (not just the male) to feel comfortable and increase arousal is for both to be actively involved in giving and receiving sensual and sexual stimulation. Do not worry about erections, focus on pleasure. Break the vicious cycle of sexual performance by focusing on receptiveness and responsiveness to pleasure; be aware of subjective arousal (feeling "turned on").

The couple can develop a giving, caring, sexually enhancing relationship. Positive anticipation, involvement, intimacy, nondemand pleasuring, and erotic scenarios and techniques (especially multiple stimulation) counteract fears, anxieties, and worries.

Non-genital and genital exercises involve sharing in a non-demanding, non-goal-oriented manner. You can extend this approach to eroticism, arousal, and erections.

An erection is a psychophysiological response that is the natural consequence of comfort, pleasure, genital stimulation, eroticism, and arousal. Sexual arousal leading to erection is the natural outcome of positive emotions and the man's being in touch with his own and his partner's sexual responsivity.

Terry and Robin

Terry and Robin were feeling very discouraged about Terry's erection problem. Previous attempts to find help had resulted in a run-around. After nine months of increasing difficulty maintaining an erection, they consulted their minister, who referred them to an internist, who saw Terry alone and immediately prescribed Viagra. Terry was not given any sexual therapy or relationship suggestions. He clung only to the hope that Viagra would work as well for him as for Bob Dole, but it did not. The internist then referred Terry to an endocrinologist. The endocrinologist tested Terry for testosterone, which proved to be in the normal range. Nonetheless, the endocrinologist gave him a testosterone injection to see if it would help. It made Terry more sexually agitated and frustrated, and his irritability created more conflict with Robin. Terry was then referred to a urologist who monitored

Terry's erections for two nights in a sleep laboratory. He suggested penile injections, which resulted in firm erections, but Terry disliked the injection process. Robin objected that the penis felt cold and mechanical, which was a turn-off for her. In addition, intercourse was painful. The urologist determined Terry's problem to be chronic, with penile prosthesis surgery the only lasting solution.

The medical process dragged out over a sixteen-month period. Meanwhile Terry's erectile dysfunction was becoming worse. He had difficulty getting erections with Robin, although he had erections on waking and when he masturbated. Erection problems seldom remain at a plateau; if there is not a positive change, anticipatory and performance anxiety grow, and erections shrink. Terry became increasingly more discouraged, and Robin felt frustrated and unsure of her sexual desirability (the woman blaming herself is neither a valid conclusion nor a helpful response). In retrospect, since Terry could get erections on waking, by masturbation, and during oral sex, it should have signaled that an extensive medical evaluation was unnecessary. Only when the man is unable to get an erection under any circumstances is a comprehensive medical evaluation necessary.

A key element in regaining erectile confidence is to reestablish comfort with desire, sensuality and touching. Both Robin and Terry had ceased to anticipate being sexual. For three years their sexual activity had been tension-filled. They still valued their intimate bond and enjoyed sharing affection. However, as soon as there was nudity, genital touching, or incipient arousal, a curtain of anxiety came down.

The sex therapy strategy to reverse this self-defeating trend began with a week of non-genital, nondemand touching in the nude both inside and outside the bedroom. Robin was actively involved in both the assessment and treatment of Terry's condition, a fact that relieved Terry and energized her. Robin had not been invited to any of the medical appointments. If Terry became aroused by their mutual touching, he was to be aware of the sensations and enjoy them but not move toward intercourse. He and Robin were pleasantly surprised to find his erections began to return. They would naturally wane, but with continued touching he would become erect again.

In introducing genital touching exercises, Robin was told to refrain from penile stimulation until Terry was comfortable and receptive. She began with sensual stimulation, playfully and seductively stroking his inner thighs, scratching his pubic hair, and with one or two fingers lightly playing with his penis. Robin found genital touching pleasurable. Terry, however, could not let go and continued to be a spectator of his penis' performance. As soon as there was the beginning of an erection, he wanted to jump into action. Rather than castigating Terry, the exercise was modified. Terry was instructed to be active in touching and stroking Robin and focus on sexual fantasies to counter his acting like a spectator. Robin stimulated him until he had an erection, and then ceased stimulation. Both became comfortable with the waxing and waning of erections.

As pleasure and eroticism increased, so did erections. The last stumbling block was for Terry to experience intercourse as a natural continuation of the pleasuring process rather than as the ultimate test of sex and masculinity. There were setbacks in this process, but it was clear they were over the hump. Both were looking forward to sex undistracted by performance fears. When his erection was not firm enough for intercourse they made the transition to a sensual scenario or an erotic, non-intercourse scenario. Reintroduction of intercourse was at Robin's initiative and she guided Terry's penis into her vagina. Terry valued Robin as his intimate sexual friend and spouse, not someone he had to perform for.

Medical Interventions
as an Additional Resource

Viagra, introduced in 1998, is a good drug. It is the first user-friendly medical intervention, much superior to injections, external pumps, and penile prostheses. In the coming years, it is likely other, more efficacious oral medications will be introduced.

The issue is how to integrate Viagra into the couple's lovemaking style. The unhelpful approach is the attempt of the male to revert back to his twenties and thirties, when he had a totally predictable and autonomous erection and his partner had no role other than to be there. The guidelines of intimacy, pleasuring, and eroticism remain valid—sexuality involves the couple sharing arousal, erection, and intercourse. Intercourse is a part of the pleasuring process—not apart from it.

Viagra is both an efficacious resource to increase blood flow to the penis and a psychological resource to combat self-consciousness and increase erectile confidence. Rather than moving to intercourse as soon as the male is erect, the couple has the freedom to enhance pleasure and eroticism and make the transition to intercourse at high levels of arousal.

Bob Dole has become the spokesman for males who have major vascular or neurological impediments that make erectile functioning impossible. For them, Viagra is a godsend, and they use it each time they engage in sex. For the majority of males, Viagra is used only occasionally, as a resource to promote erectile confidence and ensure against relapse.

First Set of Exercises: Waxing and Waning

Begin by sitting, holding hands, and discussing how you felt and what you learned in the non-genital and genital pleasuring exercises. What are your personal or couple sexual traps when it comes to erections? How can you avoid falling into them? Be an intimate team; enjoy giving and receiving pleasure.

Proceed to a relaxing, sensuous shower. Wash each other, including genitals; rub and pat your partner dry. Use a comfortable pleasuring position. Let the woman be pleasure-giver, beginning with non-genital touching. The man accepts feelings of pleasure and is receptive and responsive as she engages in playful, seductive touching of his inner thighs, scrotum, perineum, and perhaps, with a finger or two, the shaft or glans of his penis. When there is penile response, she can move to stroking and caressing his penis while continuing a variety of additional pleasuring techniques. Penile stimulation is not pleasurable or erotic until there is at least a moderate amount of arousal.

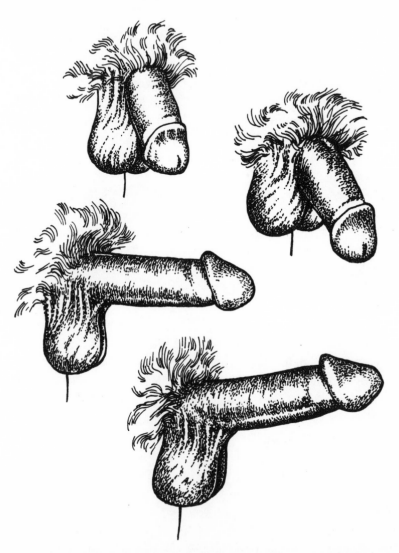

External male genitalia in the sexual response cycle: from nonstimulated state to early excitement phase to excitement plateau to orgasmic phase.

To avoid being a passive, obsessive spectator, the man is encouraged to touch the woman so that he keeps contact and is actively involved in pleasurable touching. When his erection grows, both partners should stop touching and lie together until his erection subsides. Be aware of feelings as the erection wanes, whether you feel anger, fright, anxiety, worry, tension, relief. When the erection has waned, the woman resumes non-genital pleasuring, then genital touching, combining pleasuring techniques which are enjoyable for her and to which he is receptive.

Instead of working to achieve an erection, the male can enjoy receiving. When an erection naturally occurs as a response to pleasurable, playful, and erotic stimulation, again cease activity until it is lost. If an erection does not occur, that is all right, too—simply proceed with the pleasuring. The focus is on accepting and enjoying touching. Enjoy sensations and feelings with no performance demand. Erections cannot be willed or forced; they are a natural response to involved, pleasurable, playful, and erotic stimulation.

The couple now switches roles, and the man, as giver, focuses on her enjoyment. He should be aware of giving pleasure and seeing her respond. Often an erection will occur naturally. Partner response and arousal are powerful aphrodisiacs. A male with erectile anxiety often falls into the pattern of viewing the woman's arousal as a threat and performance demand. Instead, he can enjoy her arousal and allow these feelings to increase his pleasure.

Do this exercise, with whatever variations you want, enough times until both partners are comfortable with achieving and losing an erection without feeling anxiety or pressure. Men are used to and prefer proceeding to intercourse on their first erection. This is a positive, sexually arousing scenario, but the couple need to develop flexible, variable sexual scenarios so they do not panic and feel dependent on his first erection. On average, the erection becomes hard and then somewhat flaccid two to five times during a forty-five-minute pleasuring period. Couples with an erection problem rush the sex and become anxious or panicky if his erection subsides. Anxiety and distraction are what cause the penis to stay soft. Worry and pressure to regain erection inhibit responsiveness, thus blocking rearousal and waxing of the erection again.

If the male is troubled by recurrent worries about losing his erection, he should focus on a sexual fantasy such as making love to an exotic woman, being caressed by four pairs of hands, or having intercourse swinging from a bell tower—any fantasy which turns him on and gets him out of the spectator role. Fantasies are a bridge to arousal, used by three out of four men during partner sex. Erotic fantasies or materials facilitate desire and arousal. They provide an erotic focus that displaces the distractions caused by anticipatory anxiety, performance anxiety, and spectatorship.

After the exercise, lie in bed and share the feelings you both experienced as the male's erection became soft and hard again. Talk about the types of stimulation that you enjoy giving and to which you are responsive. Notice the difference: you are working together rather than making demands and feeling pressure. Be aware of the decrease in anxiety and worry as you accept the naturally occurring waxing and waning of erections. Subjective arousal, feeling turned-on, usually precedes objective arousal. You are regaining comfort and confidence with arousal and erection.

Second Set of Exercises:
Playing with the Penis Around the Vagina

Begin with mutual nondemand pleasuring. When the male achieves erection, the woman continues stimulation, but this time the man should concentrate on trying to maintain the erection. Focusing on an erection almost invariably results in losing an erection. For when the man concentrates on his erection, his involvement and arousal decrease, and he becomes distracted and breaks the erotic flow. His erection dissipates and stays soft. The way to maintain arousal is to focus on feelings and sensations, accept sensual and sexual pleasure, stay involved psychologically and physically and enjoy the erotic flow. Do not become a distracted spectator.

To reinforce this point, the man should shut his partner out and focus on working to regain an erection. His penis will almost invariably remain flaccid, because psychologically and sexually he is not there. Notice the pressure and tension he puts himself under. He is not giving and receiving pleasure. Instead, he has become an isolated, distracted performer. Psychologically he is alone in bed. He is shut off from the enjoyment and involvement of intimate contact, pleasuring, give-and-take genital stimulation, and the erotic flow.

The woman, meanwhile, will be aware how sexuality has become a demanding, goal-oriented job to produce the erection as opposed to a mutual pleasuring and erotic experience. Notice how frustrated and worried she has become, and how out of touch she is with her partner as he works *alone.* Her pleasure and arousal decrease. Touching and sexuality are no longer fun, but a performance goal. Sexuality should be a positive feedback system of anticipation, comfort, pleasure, playfulness, eroticism, and arousal. But it can become a negative feedback system of anticipatory anxiety, performance anxiety, self-conscious attempts to force erection, and avoidance of sex because it is stressful and results in embarrassing failures.

The couple needs to be aware of these negativity traps. Share feelings about the difference between being together in a nondemanding atmosphere, mutual pleasuring, accepting naturally occurring responsiveness and arousal as opposed to working alone, worrying, feeling tense, being a spectator, trying to will an erection, and being goal-oriented.

This part of the exercise demonstrates the negative effects of focusing on sexual performance and erection. One demonstration is enough. Unlike other exercises, this one need not be repeated.

Return to pleasuring by using mutual nondemand touching. Be aware of the feelings and sensations of giving and receiving stimulation so each partner's comfort, pleasure, and arousal feeds the other's. When you are feeling receptive, switch to the female-on-top intercourse position. You will not be engaging in intercourse, but it is important to experience comfort (low anxiety, no pressure to perform, enjoying what you are doing) with his penis near her vagina. Make yourselves at ease, perhaps with a pillow under the man's head and she in a position to have easy access to his genitals. He can accept and enjoy her touching. If he is more responsive when actively touching and caressing, he should feel free to do so. He can guide and make specific requests. Men with erection difficulties are shy about being assertive sexually—this is your time to break that pattern.

The woman can massage his arms and chest; she can run her fingers over his face, highlighting his features. She can massage his genital area, beginning with his inner thighs, working up and over his penis and pubic hair, over the stomach, and back again in a rhythmic movement. When he gets an erection as a natural outcome of feeling pleasure and accepting erotic stimulation, she ceases activity until his erection becomes soft. This is a natural result of stopping touching; neither partner should feel worried or panicky. His erection might wax and wane two to five times. Although most males prefer to go to intercourse and orgasm on their first erection (the pattern they learned in initial sexual experiences), it is freeing to realize you can become comfortable and confident with the waning and waxing of erections. The female returns to pleasuring and he makes requests and guides. As receptivity and arousal increase, erection will naturally occur again.

She takes his penis in her hand, gently caressing and rubbing it around her vulva. Rub his penis on her mons, clitoral shaft, labia, and close to (but not into) her vagina. If at any point you notice your partner becoming tense or anxious, continue caressing but move back a step until both of you are feeling comfortable. Resume penile-vulva stimulation when your partner again feels open and receptive. Repeat this sequence with the man again achieving erection with his penis around her vulva, allowing it to become soft, and remaining open to pleasurable and erotic stimulation.

You might do this exercise just once or repeat it several times with variations of position and stimulation until both people feel comfortable with the penis around the labia, clitoris, and vagina. Remember, in a typical pleasuring process the erection will not always remain "hard"; it is normal for his erection to wax and wane.

End the exercise either with the woman being the recipient or using mutual stimulation whereby you enjoy giving to each other. It is important for her to be involved. She should feel the appreciation and caring in the man's gestures, words, and stimulation. There is a world of difference between "giving pleasure" and "mechanically doing" the partner as compensation for an erection problem. Both can enjoy manual, oral, or rubbing stimulation to orgasm. Even after you have re-introduced intercourse, be open to both sensual scenarios and erotic, non-intercourse scenarios as back-ups.

Third Set of Exercises: Comfort, Pleasure, Eroticism, Arousal, Erection, Intercourse

Enjoy mutual pleasuring and a sense of receptivity and responsivity, then move to the female-on-top intercourse position. From this position the woman can use a variety of pleasuring techniques; enjoy playing and teasing. The woman can rub her partner's penis around her labia and clitoris, against her thigh, around her vagina. Both should be aware of her enjoyment and responsiveness, which include, but are not limited to, his penis. He is aware of his arousal as well as hers. The natural result of pleasure, eroticism, and arousal is erection.

At the woman's initiative, the penis should be inserted into the vagina. The man is not responsible for pushing or directing; the initiative and timing rests with her. If she notices tension increasing or his penis becoming soft, she can modify her stimulation until both are feeling receptive.

The woman can insert the penis by leaning back at a forty-five degree angle so it easily enters the vagina. She can guide insertion with her hand on his penis. If there is tension or feeling of forced action, cease intromission and return to pleasuring. Intromission is part of the pleasuring and arousal process, not a pass-fail test. Be aware that a "rock-hard" erection is not necessary for intromission. Intercourse is preferable with varying levels of firmness.

The woman directs slow, rhythmic thrusting. The tendency is to force thrusting or make it rapid in order to maintain arousal. Slow, rhythmic thrusting can better facilitate arousal and erection because it allows the male to focus on pleasurable movement and an awareness of vaginal warmth and wetness. Continue giving and receiving multiple stimulation during intercourse to heighten involvement and arousal.

If desired, continue to orgasm. Orgasm occurs as a natural consequence of sexual arousal and going with the erotic flow; it need not be striven for or forced. Sex should not end abruptly after orgasm. Orgasm is not the end of sexual feelings and responsiveness. Afterplay is as much an integral part of sexual activity as is pleasuring. This is true whether the scenario involves intercourse or erotic, non-intercourse sex.

He will lose part of his erection shortly after ejaculation. This is part of the natural physiological resolution process. Some couples enjoy maintaining the intercourse position, and continue caressing, holding, and talking. Others prefer to disengage, touch in a different position, and share feelings. Examples of afterplay positions include sitting facing each other, lying side by side, the man lying on his back and the woman laying her head on his shoulder, the spoon position in which her back lies against his chest and his arms encompass her. Many couples prefer to wash the semen off, others would rather just lie there. Find what is most comfortable and sensual; share your preferences. Feel comfortable with afterplay, the natural culmination of a sexual experience. You have shared an intense physical experience; share coming down together.

Fourth Set of Exercises:
Integrating Arousal and Intercourse

You have come a long way in sharing pleasure, feeling comfortable with sexual expression, and experiencing erections as a natural step in the process of receptivity, responsivity, and arousal. During this set of exercises experiment with scenarios and techniques so that comfort and confidence with erections are robust.

Begin pleasuring in a position you both enjoy. When you are feeling receptive, the woman can rub her partner's penis (whether flaccid, semi-erect, or erect) against her vulva while at the same time the man uses his fingers to caress her clitoral shaft and labia. In the process of giving pleasure and attending to her feelings, the man becomes aroused and an erection develops naturally. The most common stimulus for his arousal is response to her arousal—an example of the "give to get" guideline. Be aware she can respond to manual, oral, rubbing, and penile (whether flaccid, semi-erect, or erect) stimulation. An erect penis is not necessary for female arousal and orgasm.

A man with erectile anxiety often avoids initiating sex because he is not sure he will be able to follow through and complete intercourse. Nor does he welcome her initiation, because he views it as a demand for a sexual performance that he is not certain he can meet. Both people can learn to accept that not every sexual experience needs to end in intercourse. Flexibility and variability can enhance sexual desire, not inhibit it. Manual, oral, rubbing, and penile stimulation are all normal techniques for meeting your partner's sexual needs as well as your own. Some women feel they must have an orgasm during intercourse; this puts tremendous pressure on the man which exacerbates erectile problems. In truth, the majority of women find it easier to be orgasmic with manual or oral stimulation. Orgasm achieved by erotic, non-intercourse stimulation is enjoyable and fulfilling.

A full erection is not necessary for vaginal intromission. If the man lies on his side and the woman lies on her back, leaning slightly toward and facing him, she can insert his penis. He should not try to force or take the initiative; rather, he should relax, accept her initiative, and continue to be actively involved in pleasuring. The woman takes his penis with both hands and inserts it into her vagina, using pelvic movements to facilitate intromission. He can kiss, caress, and fondle while accepting her stimulation. Frequently, after intromission or during thrusting, his arousal increases and his erection becomes firmer.

If there are problems with intromission, the woman can be active in providing stimulation and facilitating intromission. Insertion can be tried from the female-on-top or another position she is comfortable with.

When he feels anxious, the male often panics and tries to force the penis into her vagina. This results in his penis becoming flaccid, causes his partner discomfort, and frustrates the couple. Performance anxiety causes people to react in self-defeating ways. If he feels anxious, he can verbalize that and request what he needs to get out of the role of the anxious spectator and become actively involved in the sexual give-and-take. He might ask her to engage in fellatio right before intromission or to stroke his testicles while fondling his penis. He might suggest standing or kneeling and facing each other to engage in mutual stimulation. He might give to her, since her arousal will build his arousal. He can request whatever will increase receptivity and responsiveness. What neither he nor she should do is stop and avoid sexual contact. If anxiety persists, they should move to nondemand, sensual touching. They can end the encounter in this sensual way, or if one of them is desirous for erotic sex, he or she can utilize manual or oral stimulation to orgasm for one or both.

Experiment with other intercourse positions. Allow the stimulation to be mutual and erotic. Remember the "give to get" guideline. Enjoy each other's sexuality and arousal without worrying or being distracted by the state of his penis. Allow stimulation to be slow, tender, caring, rhythmic, flowing. Do not try to hurry or force arousal. An involved, aroused partner is the best facilitator of arousal and erection. Let intromission be a naturally occurring event rather than a major hurdle; intercourse is a continuation of the pleasuring process, not a pass-fail test.

The man can initiate and guide intromission. If he becomes anxious or tries to force intercourse, he can move a step back, and she can initiate and guide intromission. Intercourse is a mutual pleasuring activity, not a goal to be achieved. Be aware of each other's feelings and continue to be caring, supportive, and giving during intercourse. Spend time in afterplay and share feelings of closeness and intimacy. Afterplay is integral to the sexual experience.

Arousal and Erection Guidelines

These guidelines can enhance arousal and erection and prevent relapse.

1. By age forty, 90 percent of males experience at least one erectile failure; this is a normal occurrence, not a sign of an erectile dysfunction.
2. The majority of erectile problems (especially for men under fifty) are caused primarily by psychological or relationship factors, not

medical or physiological malfunctions. To comprehensively evaluate medical factors, including side effects of medication, consult a urologist with training in erectile dysfunction.

3. Erectile problems can be caused by a wide variety of factors including alcohol, anxiety, depression, vascular or neurological deficits, distraction, anger, side effects of medication, frustration, hormonal deficiency, fatigue, not feeling sexual at that time or with that partner. As men age, the hormonal, vascular and neurological systems become less efficient so psychological, relational, and erotic factors become more important.

4. Medical interventions, especially the oral medication, Viagra, can be a valuable resource to facilitate erectile function, but it is not a "magic pill." The couple need to integrate Viagra (or other medical interventions) into their lovemaking style.

5. Do not believe the myth of the "male machine, ready to have intercourse at any time, with any woman, in any situation." You and your penis are human. You are not a performance machine.

6. View the erectile difficulty as a situational problem, do not overreact and label yourself "impotent" or put yourself down as a "failure."

7. A pervasive myth holds that if a man loses his initial erection, it means he is sexually turned off. It is a natural physiological process for erections to wax and wane during prolonged pleasuring.

8. In a forty-five-minute pleasuring session, erections will wax and wane two to five times. Subsequent erections, intercourse, and orgasm are quite satisfying.

9. You do not need an erect penis to satisfy a woman. Orgasm can be achieved through manual, oral, or rubbing stimulation. If you have difficulty getting or maintaining an erection, do not stop the sexual interaction. Women find it arousing to have their partner's fingers, tongue, or penis (erect or flaccid) used for stimulation.

10. Actively involve yourself in giving and receiving pleasurable and erotic touching. Erection is a natural result of pleasure, feeling turned-on, and eroticism.

11. You cannot will or force an erection. Do not be a passive "spectator" who is distracted by the state of his penis. Sex is not a spectator sport, it requires active involvement.

12. Allow the woman to initiate intercourse and guide your penis into her vagina. This reduces performance pressure, and since she is the expert on her vagina, is the most practical procedure.

13. Feel comfortable saying, "I want sex to be pleasurable and playful. When I feel pressure to perform, I get uptight and sex is not good. We can make sexuality enjoyable by taking it at a comfortable pace, playing and pleasuring, and being an intimate team."

14. Erectile problems do not affect the ability to ejaculate (men can ejaculate with a flaccid penis). The male relearns to ejaculate to the cue of an erect penis.

15. One way to regain confidence is through masturbation. During masturbation you can practice gaining and losing erections, relearn ejaculating with an erection, and focus on fantasies and stimulation which transfer to partner sex.

16. Do not try to use a waking erection for quick intercourse. This erection is associated with REM sleep and results from dreaming and being close to the partner. Men vainly try to have intercourse with their morning erection before losing it. Remember, arousal and erection are regainable. Morning is a good time to be sexual.

17. When sleeping, you have an erection every ninety minutes—three to five erections a night. Sex is a natural physiological function. Do not block it by anticipatory anxiety, performance anxiety, distraction, or putting yourself down. Give yourself (and your partner) permission to enjoy the pleasure of sexuality.

18. Make clear, direct, assertive requests (not demands) for stimulation you find erotic. Verbally and nonverbally guide your partner in how to pleasure and arouse you.

19. Stimulating a flaccid penis is counterproductive. The man becomes distracted and obsessed about the state of his penis. Engage in sensuous, playful, nondemand touching. Enjoy giving and receiving stimulation rather than trying to "will an erection."

20. Attitudes and self-thoughts affect arousal. The key is "sex and pleasure" not "sex and performance."

21. A sexual experience is best measured by pleasure and satisfaction, not whether you had an erection, how hard it was, or whether your partner was orgasmic. Some sexual experiences will be great for both, some better for one than the other, some unremarkable, and others unsuccessful. Do not put your sexual self-esteem on the line at each sexual experience.

Closing Thoughts

Be comfortable facilitating each other's responsiveness, which naturally leads to arousal and erection. Anticipatory anxiety, performance anxiety, being in the spectator role, feelings of frustration and blaming are thereby minimized.

Does this mean you will never have an experience of not getting or losing an erection? Realistically, you will experience erectile difficulties from time to time. Most men do. On occasions of fatigue, anxiety over money or work, little sexual desire, interruptions, stress, or feeling distracted, you will be less responsive. You might not get an erection, or not have an erection firm enough for intercourse. That does not mean you have an erectile dysfunction, unless you again fall into the performance anxiety or distracted spectator trap. What it means is that at this point, in this situation, you are not feeling sexually responsive or aroused enough for intercourse. You can decide not to have sex that day; use manual, oral, or rubbing stimulation to orgasm; relax and enjoy the sensual give-and-take; give to your partner; or have your partner guide intromission with a semi-erection. Be aware you have alternatives for a positive sensual and/or erotic experience. There is no need to feel worried or panicky. As long as you do not fall into the traps of performance anxiety, playing the spectator role, or trying to force an erection, you will have a pleasurable, satisfying sexual relationship.

You can continue to enjoy the intimacy and mutual responsiveness that afford you comfort with sensuality, eroticism, arousal, erections, and intercourse. Enjoy sexual experiences which include, but are not limited to, intercourse.

19

——

Letting Go:
Overcoming Ejaculatory Inhibition

The problem of women not reaching orgasm has been widely discussed by sex researchers and therapists, but scant attention has been paid to the equivalent problem for men. Many human sexuality books omit discussion of this particular sexual dysfunction, the male's inability to reach orgasm during partner sex. When it is mentioned, the terms used—"retarded ejaculation" or "ejaculatory incompetence"—have a derogatory connotation. We prefer the term "ejaculatory inhibition" because it best describes the sexual problem without negative connotations.

Ejaculatory inhibition has been viewed as a rare and difficult to understand dysfunction. Research on ejaculatory inhibition finds that in its most severe form, the total inability to ejaculate, it is extremely rare. Not being able to ejaculate intravaginally is more common, often coming to the sex therapist's attention because the couple now want to become pregnant. Ejaculatory inhibition is most common in its intermittent form and affects as many as 15 percent of males at some time in their lives, especially after forty.

It is the man's psychological and sexual inhibitions that interfere with the natural pattern of sexual arousal resulting in orgasm. Inability to ejaculate or difficulty ejaculating stems from some type of inhibition—beginning intercourse at low levels of arousal, the inability to let go, being emotionally uninvolved, fear of pregnancy, inability to communicate with and make requests of your partner.

The most frequent pattern is intermittent ejaculatory inhibition, in which a man who had regularly ejaculated begins to have difficulty reaching orgasm, especially during intercourse. If not discussed and dealt with, ejaculatory problems become progressively more severe and chronic. The second most common pattern involves males who reach orgasm with a specific type of stimulation (rubbing against bed-sheets or the partner's thigh, manual or oral stimulation, or a fetish arousal pattern), but not during intercourse.

Ejaculatory inhibition is different from the normal aging physio-logical process of a lessened need to ejaculate at each sexual en-counter. With ejaculatory inhibition the male desires to ejaculate, but has great difficulty or is unable to do so. Ejaculatory inhibition can af-fect males in their twenties, but is most prevalent among men after forty and especially after fifty. Ejaculation and orgasm are not the same phenomena, although the terms are used interchangeably. For example, most males develop retrograde ejaculation after prostate surgery, i.e., he is orgasmic, but he ejaculates into the bladder rather than out through the penis. If there are medical or physiological con-cerns (especially side effects of medication), consult a urologist.

There are a number of inhibitions which can cause this dys-function, including anger at the partner, lack of effective sexual stim-ulation, shutting oneself off from sexual involvement, beginning intercourse before feeling aroused, performance anxiety, sexual guilt, low subjective arousal even though the male has a firm erection, shy-ness about requesting multiple stimulation, and a man putting his partner's sexual needs before his own. Sex is a cooperative, sharing interaction between two people who are actively involved in giving and receiving pleasure. This process is blocked for the man with ejacula-tory inhibition.

Sexual functioning includes desire, arousal, orgasm, and emotional satisfaction. With ejaculatory inhibition the natural cycle of antici-pating sex, responding to stimulation with arousal which naturally culminates in orgasm, is disrupted. The man (and his partner) will push hard to reach orgasm so even if he manages to "come," neither intercourse nor orgasm holds much pleasure for him. Rather than orgasm being the natural culmination of an arousing sexual experience, it becomes an anxiety-provoking goal he often fails to achieve. When he does reach orgasm it is more a relief than a pleasure.

Ejaculatory Inhibition as a Couple Problem

As with other sexual difficulties, ejaculatory inhibition is best thought of as a couple problem. The couple needs to see it as "their" problem, not "his" problem. It is the couple, not just the man, that has to increase stimulation and allow arousal to naturally flow to orgasm. A comfortable, involved, sexually giving partner is essential. A particular trap is the belief that a "real man" does not need the woman's involvement and stimulation to reach orgasm. The man mistakenly thinks he *should* be able to do it himself without making requests of her. He believes the myth that only "wimps" discuss sexual needs or feelings. As a man begins the aging process (in his thirties and continuing throughout the life span), he benefits from a sharing, intimate sexual relationship.

Development of Ejaculatory Inhibition

There are three major forms of ejaculatory inhibition, but they have myriad variations and individual differences. The first type includes men who have difficulty from the beginning of their sexual lives. While the great majority of these men do ejaculate during masturbation, some of them develop either an idiosyncratic arousal pattern or a fetish pattern that is not transferable to partner sex. Such men thus find it difficult or impossible to ejaculate with a partner. We urge those males to seek professional sex therapy. Although the exercises might be helpful, it is doubtful these alone will be sufficient to change ejaculatory inhibition. Ejaculatory inhibition is changeable for a motivated couple working with a competent sex therapist.

A second pattern emerges with men who experience orgasm with manual, oral, or rubbing stimulation, but are unable to ejaculate during intercourse or have great difficulty doing so. Some men lose arousal during intercourse and in turn lose the erection; others maintain arousal and erection for over twenty minutes (and some for an hour or more), but are not able to let go and be orgasmic. The therapeutic strategy in these cases is to identify the man's inhibitions and fears and to develop sexual scenarios and techniques to overcome them, because commonly the male is embarrassed to ask for multiple stimulation during intercourse.

The third form of ejaculatory inhibition, and the most common, involves men who have a history of orgasm during intercourse and then develop an intermittent problem. For some men this affects only orgasm, while for others it affects the entire spectrum of desire, arousal and orgasm. This problem can remain intermittent, but it often becomes pervasive and chronic. Although sometimes only ejaculation is affected, it can cause erectile dysfunction, which leads to inhibited sexual desire and sexual avoidance.

In summary, ejaculatory inhibition is neither rare nor impossible to treat. It is prevalent, has many variations, and is a complex but understandable dysfunction. Most important, it is changeable. The couple can identify and overcome inhibitions; increase comfort, eroticism, and arousal; and gain confidence that arousal will regularly culminate in orgasm.

Leo and Alix

Leo's experience is instructive. As a young man, the only times he had problems with ejaculation were the first one or two intercourse encounters with a new partner. After overcoming his initial anxiety, Leo had no difficulty reaching orgasm. Leo had begun masturbating at age twelve, and masturbated once or twice a day. This pattern is well within the normal range for adolescent males, except that Leo experienced a strong mixture of excitement, guilt, and anxiety during masturbation. His fantasies focused obsessively on the woman stroking his penis very hard, using a leather glove. Initially, he had experimented with a number of fantasies, but since fifteen he had obsessively and exclusively employed the leather glove fantasy (this is an example of a fetish arousal).

Initially, Leo found partner sex exciting. He married Alix at twenty-four and sex went well for a year and a half. Then he began having occasional difficulties reaching orgasm. When Alix asked what the problem was or if there was any way she could help, he told her the problem was in *her* mind.

When they came for therapy, Leo and Alix had been married eighteen years. Alix blamed their sexual problems on Leo's loss of erection during intercourse and his low sexual interest. Alix was frustrated and depressed, at her "wit's end." Leo was an evasive, reluctant client. In careful questioning during the individual sex history, it became clear Leo could function fine and had a high sex interest, as evidenced by daily masturbation to his glove fantasy. Leo was embarrassed by his fetish arousal pattern and wanted it to remain secret. He did not understand that much of Alix's frustration centered on her feeling that Leo did not communicate honestly.

With the therapist's help, Leo's "sexual secret" was disclosed. This allowed Leo and Alix to deal constructively with issues of desire, arousal, and orgasm. Leo confronted the embarrassment, confusion, and guilt over his driven, yet inhibiting, fetish pattern. The therapist helped Alix deal with her anger at being misled.

The sexual problem was redefined as ejaculatory inhibition, with the goal of increasing couple involvement, eroticism, and arousal. Leo agreed to masturbate only when Alix was not at home and/or not interested in being sexual. Leo was strongly encouraged to expand his repertoire of sexual fantasies and to approach masturbation in a guilt-free, comfortable manner. He had to dramatically alter his fetish pattern if partner sex was to be successful. In couple experiences, Leo was not to retreat into the glove fantasy. He was to be an active, involved sexual participant. Leo was receptive and responsive to Alix's manual stimulation. They did not proceed to intercourse until Leo was highly aroused. During intercourse he was assertive in making requests, especially for multiple stimulation. He increased the rhythm of coital thrusting, asked Alix to stimulate his testicles, and enjoyed stroking her breasts as he approached orgasm. Alix found this new involvement and multiple stimulation quite arousing, which in turn increased Leo's arousal. The best aphrodisiac is an involved, aroused partner.

Building Sexual Intimacy

Leo and Alix illustrate the importance of working as an intimate team in treating ejaculatory inhibition. Verbal and physical intimacy breaks down the walls of inhibition and sexual isolation. Mutual involvement in the give-and-take of erotic sex is key in overcoming ejaculatory inhibition. Treatment can be conceptualized as a one-two-three combination—being an intimate sexual team, increasing comfort with nondemand pleasuring, and increasing arousal through erotic stimulation. Even more important than mastering sexual techniques are making changes in attitudes and being emotionally involved and letting go.

Shared intimacy and increasing sexual give and take is new for couples in which the man has a history of ejaculatory inhibition. He has been emotionally isolated and resents the lack of effective stimulation, although he is unable to request it. The woman falls into a passive, frustrated, and ineffective sexual pattern. Increased involvement and intimacy are new for her also. Each partner holds the personal responsibility for sexuality and each is part of an intimate team committed to effecting change. Both need to lean to share sexual feelings, requests, turn-ons, and erotic scenarios and techniques.

First Set of Exercises: Sexual Involvement

Talk over a glass of wine or cup of tea and renew your commitment to work together in order to revitalize sexual expression, especially by increasing eroticism and arousal. Focus on the present and future; put aside the anxiety, guilt, frustration, and embarrassment of the past.

Take a bath or shower and use that time to share feelings, increase contact, and use touch as play in this nondemanding situation. When you go into the bedroom, utilize touching you have learned from the

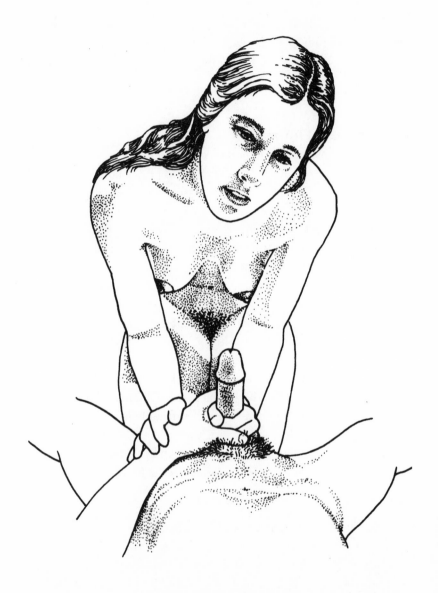

Building sexual intimacy through erotic stimulation of the male
by his partner.

non-genital and genital pleasuring exercises as they enhance receptivity and responsivity. Be aware of touching and being touched; enjoy sharing pleasure.

Move to the position where the man is lying on his back, perhaps with a pillow under his head, and the woman is sitting next to him with his legs over hers—a comfortable position for her to stroke his body, especially his genitals. It also enables partners to maintain good eye contact and gives the man easy access to the woman's thighs and breasts. She can provide a range of stimulation to his penis, scrotum, inner thighs, perineum, and anal area. At the same time, she can touch his chest, stomach, neck, legs, and feet. Experiment with intermixing oral, manual, and rubbing stimulation. Allow touching to be slow, tender, rhythmic, caring, and flowing. He can experiment with keeping his eyes open or closed, being passive or stroking her as she touches him, being silent or talking. Break down walls and inhibitions and really be there with each other. Let him become aware of what he needs to feel sexually and emotionally involved. Does sharing sexual feelings and fantasies facilitate or inhibit arousal? During this exercise, keep a prohibition on orgasm so you can focus on feelings of involvement, pleasure, eroticism and arousal.

End the exercise with mutual touching and caressing. Afterward, talk clearly and directly about what you can do to increase involvement, eroticism, and arousal so sexuality is a shared pleasure.

Second Set of Exercises:
Requesting Multiple Stimulation

The man can choose the position which is most involving for him and allows free expression of his sexual feelings. He might use a position from a previous exercise, kneel over her so she can stroke him while he stimulates her and rubs his penis against her breast, or stand in front of a mirror where visual stimulation adds an erotic dimension. As pleasuring proceeds, make at least two sexual requests to heighten arousal. The requests can be verbal or conveyed by guiding her with your hand, moving your body toward her so you get the stimulation you want, or moving her head, mouth, or hand. You have a perfect right to make sexual requests. Your request might be to stimulate her because your arousal increases as her arousal grows. You could orally stimulate her breasts or vulva, rub your penis between her legs or breasts, stimulate her breast and anal area while she is giving penile stimulation, or move your penis in rhythm with her pelvic movements. You might request that she verbalize her feelings, share a sexual fantasy, or tell you how turned on she feels when you touch her. She should be open to such requests, but should not feel pressure to do something which is a turn-off for her. Remember, these are requests—not demands. The woman is responsible for herself sexually, as is the man.

You can lift the prohibition on orgasm. This does not mean setting a performance demand to have an orgasm. Feel as much arousal as you can and go with the erotic flow. Make requests for multiple stimulation, which can include touching, switching positions, being stimulated, utilizing a range of sensory modalities—movement, sight, smell, touch, and hearing. Use sexual fantasies to increase arousal. Most males employ sexual fantasies during partner sex. If sharing fantasies increases your arousal, feel free to use them. Fantasies serve as a bridge to increase arousal, not as a wall to isolate you sexually. Be open to an orgasmic experience for one or both. Remember, orgasm is a natural result of increasing sexual involvement and arousal, not an isolated performance goal. Afterward, discuss the sexual requests and multiple stimulation techniques you enjoy and how to integrate these into your future sexual experience as a couple.

Third Set of Exercises: Orgasm Triggers

Most men who experience ejaculatory inhibition have no trouble being orgasmic during masturbation. Major reasons are comfort and the confidence that arousal will naturally flow to orgasm. Stimulation and arousal are under the man's control and therefore predictable; he is not self-conscious. Being orgasmic is expected; it is a habit. The man has a sense of control over his readiness to let go. He knows his "orgasm triggers" and is not self-conscious in utilizing them.

In this exercise, you will share your orgasm triggers during partner sex. When approaching orgasm, some men increase muscle tension by stretching their legs or curling their toes; others make sounds or breathe loudly and rapidly as they let go; some increase pelvic thrusting; others verbalize they are "going to come"; some imagine the culmination of their sexual fantasy and orgasm in reality as they fantasize orgasm. What are your orgasm triggers? Share these with your partner before beginning. Verbalizing has a disinhibiting effect, making it easier to let go and use orgasm triggers during the sexual experience.

Allow arousal and turn-ons to build; enjoy the erotic flow. Let sexual requests and multiple stimulation flow smoothly. Some men find it easier to be orgasmic with manual, oral, or rubbing stimulation, but others find intercourse easier and their preferred mode to share orgasm. Use the intercourse position where you are most sexually expressive. Males prefer man-on-top or rear entry, although woman-on-top and the side-by-side position have gained popularity because they facilitate multiple stimulation. Multiple stimulation is not just for pleasuring; it is equally erotic during intercourse.

Do not rush sensual and sexual pleasuring. Too many males prematurely initiate intercourse just as they start becoming aroused or when they sense their partner is ready. Be selfish. Let arousal build. Delay intromission until you are feeling highly aroused. Be sure subjective arousal is as strong as your erection. Allow yourself to be involved throughout intercourse; use the type and rhythm of movement which is most arousing. Some males prefer slow instead of rapid thrusting, others prefer circular movement to in-out or up-down. Request and engage in multiple stimulation during intercourse. Focus on your orgasm triggers and let go. Do not let anything inhibit or block your arousal, especially self-consciousness or feeling it is "not right."

If it is easier to let go and use your orgasm triggers during erotic, non-intercourse sex, feel free to switch stimulation and position. Many men have their first orgasmic experience during self-stimulation with their partner present. She holding or caressing you during self-stimulation can enhance sexual feelings. Once you are comfortable and confident being orgasmic during manual, oral, or rubbing stimulation, you can practice being orgasmic with intercourse. Continue stimulation until you feel almost at the point of orgasm, and then initiate intercourse. Use thrusting and multiple stimulation to heighten arousal and facilitate letting go and ejaculating.

End this exercise in a manner that is pleasurable for both people. You have focused on feelings of arousal and letting go; now mutually feel the warmth and caring of being together in afterplay.

Fourth Set of Exercises:
Multiple Stimulation During Intercourse

Why should multiple stimulation cease because intercourse begins? Males mistakenly believe a "real man" needs nothing more than thrusting into a wet vagina to reach orgasm. For some men, some of the time, that is true. Yet many men, especially as they age, want and need multiple stimulation.

The most common form of multiple stimulation is use of fantasy. Approximately 75 percent of males utilize fantasy during intercourse. Fantasies serve as a bridge to heighten arousal. Do not worry if your fantasies are "strange" and have nothing to do with your partner; that is the nature of erotic fantasies. Sexual fantasies are socially undesirable, as they involve being sexual with "forbidden" partners who use "kinky" techniques in bizarre positions or circumstances. This does *not* mean these are your true sexual desires. Fantasy and behavior are very different realms. The exotic "forbidden fruit" aspect of fantasies is what makes them erotic. Enjoy fantasies for what they are, a bridge to increased arousal during partner sex. Fantasies are only problematic when the man becomes obsessive or uses them to isolate himself and block interaction with his partner. Use fantasies as a bridge to arousal, not as a wall to block partner involvement.

Use the intercourse position which allows you the most expressiveness and eroticism. Use a common position or try a position where you kneel on pillows (both for comfort and so your penis is equivalent to her vulva). The woman sits on a chair or bed with pillows for back support. The kneeling-sitting position was developed for late-stage pregnancy as there is no pressure on her stomach. It was adapted for treating ejaculatory inhibition because it facilitates use of multiple stimulation during intercourse and promotes freedom of movement. This position allows good eye contact and easy access to the woman's neck, breasts, vulva, and clitoris. She can stroke his chest and stomach, and has good access to his scrotum and testicles.

In this exercise the male controls coital thrusting and utilizes whatever type of intercourse movement he finds most arousing. The woman's initiation of slow extended coital thrusting might be arousing for one man while another might prefer the woman to be passive while he moves in short, rapid strokes. Many males enjoy testicle stimulation during intercourse; others prefer kissing and stroking the partner or giving or receiving anal stimulation.

No matter which intercourse position you use, be active, involved partners in giving and receiving pleasure. He needs to be aware of what stimulation, in what sequence, and with what timing is most arousing. He should feel free to make verbal and nonverbal requests. As arousal builds, focus on erotic feelings and sensations, be aware of orgasm triggers, let go and allow your arousal to naturally culminate in orgasm.

The sexual experience does not end with orgasm. Stay together to talk, stroke, and reaffirm your desire to share. Acknowledge the changes that have occurred as you break down sexual inhibitions and become a giving, intimate couple who share orgasm.

Closing Thoughts

Ejaculatory inhibition is a serious dysfunction which has been largely ignored. The challenge for the man is to break silence and isolation and ask his partner for increased sharing, intimacy, multiple stimulation, and eroticism. Sexuality is best when it combines emotional intimacy, non-demand pleasuring, and erotic stimulation both before and during intercourse. Let go and experience the joys of orgasm.

Appendix I

Choosing a Therapist

A s stated in the first chapter, this is not a do-it-yourself therapy book. Couples are reluctant to consult a therapist, feeling that to do so is a sign of "craziness," a confession of inadequacy, or an admission that their relationship is in dire straits. In reality, seeking professional help is a sign of psychological strength. Entering marital or sex therapy means you realize there is a problem and you have made a commitment to resolve the issues and promote marital and sexual growth.

The mental health field can be confusing. Marital and sex therapy are clinical subspecialties. They are offered by several groups of professionals including psychologists, social workers, marriage therapists, psychiatrists, and pastoral counselors. The professional background of the practitioner is of less importance than her or his competency in dealing with your specific problem.

Many people have health insurance that provides coverage for mental health, and they can thus afford the services of a private practitioner. Those who do not have either the financial resources or insurance could consider a city or county mental health clinic, a university or medical school mental health outpatient clinic, or a family services center. Clinics usually have a sliding fee scale (i.e., the fee is based on your ability to pay).

When choosing a therapist be assertive in asking about credentials and areas of expertise. Ask the clinician what percentage of her or his patients remain married, how long therapy can be expected to last, and whether the focus is specifically on sexual problems or more generally on communication or relationship issues. A competent therapist will be open to discussing these issues. Be especially diligent in questioning credentials, such as university degrees and licensing, and be wary of people who call themselves personal counselors, marriage counselors, or sex counselors. There are poorly qualified persons—and some outright quacks—in any field.

One of the best resources for obtaining a referral is to call a local professional organization such as a psychological association, marriage and family therapy association, mental health association, or mental health clinic. You can ask for a referral from a family physician, minister, or friend. If you are specifically interested in sex therapy, you can contact the American Association of Sex Educators, Counselors, and Therapists through the Internet at Aasect.org for their therapist referral network, or write or call for a list of certified sex therapists in your area—P.O. Box 5488, Richmond, VA 23220, 804-644-3288. You could also check the Internet site for the American Association of Marriage and Family at Therapistlocator.net.

Feel free to talk with two or three therapists before deciding on one with whom to work. Be aware of comfort with the therapist, degree of rapport, and whether the therapist's assessment of the problem and approach to treatment make sense to you. Once you begin, give therapy a chance to be helpful. There are few miracle cures. Change requires commitment and is a gradual and often difficult process. Although some benefit from short-term therapy (fewer than ten sessions), most people find the therapeutic process will take four months to a year or longer. The role of the therapist is that of a consultant rather than decision maker. Therapy requires effort, both in the session and at home. Therapy helps to change attitudes, feelings, and behavior. Therapy can make your marital and sexual life more satisfying.

Appendix II

Books for Further Reading

Butler, Robert, and Myrna Lewis. *Love and Sex After Sixty*. New York: G. K. Hall, 1996.

Ellison, Carol. *Women's Sexualities*. Oakland: New Harbinger, 2001.

Folky, Sallie, Sally Kope, and Dennis Sugrue, *Sex Matters for Women*. New York: Guilford, 2002.

Goodwin, Aurelie and Marc Agronin. *A Woman's Guide To Overcoming Sexual Fear and Pain*. Oakland: New Harbinger, 1998.

Gordon, Sol. *Why Love Is Not Enough*. Boston: Bob Adams, 1990.

Hafner, Debra. *From Diapers To Dating*. New York: Newmarket, 2000.

Heiman, Julia and Joseph LoPiccolo. *Becoming Orgasmic*. New York: Prentice-Hall, 1988.

Maltz, Wendy. *The Sexual Healing Journey*. New York: Harper-Collins, 2001.

McCarthy, Barry and Emily McCarthy. *Male Sexual Awareness*. New York: Carroll and Graf, 1988.

McCarthy, Barry and Emily McCarthy. *Couple Sexual Awareness*. New York: Carroll and Graf, 1998.

Michael, Robert, John Gagnon, Edward Laumann, and Gina Kalota. *Sex In America*. Boston: Little, Brown, 1994.

Zilbergeld, Bernie. *The New Male Sexuality*. New York: Bantam Books, 1997.

Zoldbrod, Aline. *Sex Smart*. Oakland: New Harbinger, 1998.